PLAYING WITH
MOVEMENT

How To Explore the Many Dimensions of
Physical Health and Performance

TODD HARGROVE

Playing With Movement
Copyright © 2019 Todd R. Hargrove

For information about this title or to order other books and or electronic media, contact the publisher:

Better Movement
129 NE 52nd St, Seattle, WA 91805

ISBN: 978-0-578-50261-8
Printed in the United States of America
Cover design by Dan Shafer.
Interior design by The Book Designers.
Thanks to Carolyn Silvernail for diagrams, drawings and assistance with cover design.

Disclaimer:
All forms of exercise carry some risk. Readers are advised to take full responsibility for their safety and their limits. The advice in this book is in no way intended to be a substitute for any advice provided by your doctor or other medical professional. The information in this book is true and correct to the best of the author's knowledge. However, science is always advancing, and therefore the information may become outdated or proven incorrect. The author and publisher disclaim all liability for damages caused by applying the recommendations in this book.

ACKNOWLEDGMENTS

Thanks to clients, colleagues and teachers for giving me the information, inspiration or support to write this book. In particular: Jason Silvernail, Christopher Johnson, Ben Cormack, Neil O'Connell, Nick Tuminello, Carolyn Silvernail, Tasha Stanton, Derek Griffin, Joletta Belton, Jules Mitchell, Ole Marten Salte, Lars Avenmarie, Rajam Roose, Rafe Kelly, Weston Edwards, Sigurd Mikkelsen, James Steele, Adam Bjerre, Israel Halperin, Keith Waldron, Cory Blickenstaff, Bronnie Lenox Thompson, Travis Pollen, Tim Rowland, Jarod Hall, Jarlo Ilano, Carrie Hall, Ryan Appell, Craig Liebenson, Eric Kruger, Allison Sim, Joletta Belton, Peter O'Sullivan, Kjartan Vibe Fersum, Sarah Haag, Sandy Hilton, Kieran O'Sullivan, Lorimer Moseley, David Butler, Mladen Jovanovic, Rob Gray, Paul Glazier, John Kiely, Frans Bosch, Scott Morrison, Jeremy Frisch, Jill Cook, Chris Beardsley, Nick Winkleman, Alex Hutchinson, Steve Magness, Craig Payne, Steven Pinker, Dan Dennett, Steve Novella, David Chapman, Robert Sapolsky. And many others I have forgotten!

Special thanks to Paul Ingraham, Stephan Guyenet and Greg Lehman for invaluable assistance with the draft.

And thanks to my family and friends for their love and support, especially Jemila, Juniper and Abezash.

CONTENTS

INTRODUCTION 1

CHAPTER 1: MOVEMENT HEALTH 9

The Many Dimensions of Movement Health 12

A Model for Movement Health 16

CHAPTER 2: PLAY 19

Play and Development 22

Play Defined. 27

Play is Intrinsically Motivating. 27

Play is Not Too Stressful 30

Play is Exploratory. 31

Play is Creative. 32

Play is Tinkering 33

Play Involves Risk 34

Can Humans Play Like Cheetahs? 38

CHAPTER 3: COMPLEXITY. 41

Emergence 44

A Crowd of Agents 46

Nesting: Subsystems and Supersystems 47

Adaptivity 48

Non-linearity. 49

Feedback Loops 50

Variability 52

Attractors 53

Self-Organization. 55

Complex Versus Complicated Problems 57

Constraints 59

CHAPTER 4: STRESS AND ADAPTATION. 65

Stress and Physical Challenge. 66

Emotional Stress 68

Stress and Adaptation 70

Sleep and Stress 75

Stress and Perception 76

Stress and Sport. 77

Playing with Stress. 79

CHAPTER 5: FITNESS 83

Physical Activity is Incredibly Good for You 85

Physical Activity as a Key Constraint on Health 88

Movement as a Nutrient 89

A Balanced Movement Diet 90

Recommendations from Health Groups. 90

Physical Activity Levels of Hunter-Gatherers 93

Low-Hanging Fruits. 95

Variability of Physical Activity. 96

Playing with Fitness 97

CHAPTER 6: ENVIRONMENT 101

The Context for Movement 103

Natural Environments 105

Affordances. 106

Affordances in the Modern World 108

Playing with the Environment 110

CHAPTER 7: STRUCTURE 113

Structure and Function 114

How Structure Adapts 117

Damage to Structure 118

The Disconnect Between Structural Damage and Pain 120

MRIs on People Without Pain 120

Many Orthopedic Surgeries Don't Work 123

Structure and Manual Therapy 127

Playing with Structure 129

CHAPTER 8: MOBILITY. **133**

Models of Functional Mobility 134

Using it or Losing It. 136

Mobility and Injury 138

Playing with Mobility 139

CHAPTER 9: POSTURE **145**

Dynamics of Posture 147

Posture and Pain 149

Posture and Core Strength. 154

Playing with Posture 156

CHAPTER 10: SKILL **161**

Coordination and Dexterity. 162

The Degrees of Freedom Problem 164

Levels of Motor Control 166

The Game is the Teacher 171

Exploring Movement Landscapes. 172

Functional and Non-Functional Variability 174

Perception and Action 176

The Role of Attention 178

Movement "Dysfunction" and the

Complexity of "Correction". 181

Playing with Movement Skill:

Options not Corrections 187

CHAPTER 11: PAIN 191

The Function of Pain 193

Basic Pain Physiology 194

Pain and the Brain 198

A Systemic View 201

Central and Peripheral Contributors to Pain 203

Simple Models for Complex Pain 206

Complex Problems, Wicked Problems,
and Pain Habits 208

RESOURCES 213

PICTURE AND ILLUSTRATION CREDITS 215

ABOUT THE AUTHOR 217

ENDNOTES 219

INDEX 241

INTRODUCTION

I t's a great gift to move your body in a way that feels strong, creative or skillful. We tend to celebrate cognitive feats like art and science as being the pride of the human species, but as movers we are not so shabby either. Humans are not the fastest or strongest animals, but we are unmatched in our versatility. We can do back flips, run for miles at a stretch, dance ballet, lift hundreds of pounds, do cartwheels, shoot long-range three pointers, climb trees and cliffs, throw curveballs, swim through oceans and lakes, and play the harmonica. Of course, not every human can do all these things (or even one!), but we all have the potential to develop an amazing variety of physical abilities. We are born to run, and also to walk, climb, dance and do millions of other things.

Unfortunately, modern humans are struggling with their movement health. Only a quarter of Americans meet the recommended physical activity guidelines, and this increases the risk for a long list of diseases.[1] In fact, a sedentary lifestyle has been compared to smoking in its effects on general health.[2] Chronic pain is the biggest source of physical disability in the world,[3] and metabolic disorders affect almost a third of the U.S. population.[4]

1

Although our culture continues to produce spectacular athletes, sport is becoming less of a game and more of a business. Kids get most of their movement from organized classes, not unstructured play.[5] As a result, they are specializing in sport earlier, and burning out faster.[6] Adults have "workout routines," but the experience is often exactly that - work and routine. The average exercise program is not very fun or meaningful. This is part of the reason exercise feels like a chore, and why most people don't do it with enough volume, variety, and intensity to get its beneficial effects. Everyone knows that physical activity provides the health benefits of a "miracle drug," but few get a sufficient dose. Maybe this shouldn't be surprising - branding movement as "medicine" makes it sound like something you would rather avoid.

If you are reading this book, you have probably already tried various methods to help yourself or others move better and feel better. Perhaps you have focused on training specific attributes like posture, mobility, or strength. Or maybe you have tried various treatment options for pain - physical therapy, corrective exercise, yoga, chiropractic, or even surgery. This book will help you understand why these methods have succeeded or failed, and how to make better choices in the future. Most importantly, it will help you take more control of your movement health, in a way that is personally meaningful to you, with less reliance on experts.

In other words, this book is about helping you solve movement problems, such as completing your first marathon, recovering from back pain, putting on more muscle, or improving your agility on the soccer field. These challenges are all *complex*, meaning they depend on millions of interlocking variables — muscular, skeletal, physiological, psychological, neurological, and environmental. With so many unknowns, the pathway to success will be somewhat different for each individual, and finding it will require some exploration.

Play is a natural behavior that evolved to help animals solve complex problems in the face of uncertainty. If you want to get better at a sport, find a sustainable exercise program, or even get out of pain, you will need to play with movement. This means moving in a way that is fun, exploratory, variable, intuitive, and personally meaningful. All animals develop skill, resilience, and well-rounded fitness through play, not "working out." But the mainstream approach to training and therapy is all work no play. It is focused on movements that are boring, repetitive, planned, stressful, and done only to accomplish some external goal. This stems from a reductive mindset that views the body as a machine to be "fixed," as opposed to an organic self-organizing system that adapts and learns. This causes a wide range of common problems, including:

- Pain treatments that are highly medicalized, expensive, and ineffective.
- Policing of normal patterns of posture and movement as "dysfunctions" that need to be "corrected."
- Sport training that relies heavily on repetitive and specialized drills, as opposed to varied games.
- Exercise programs that are meaningless and dispiriting.

The arguments in this book are not based on romantic feel-good reasoning, or nostalgia for sunny days at the park when we were children. They rely on a substantial body of evidence and theory pulled from diverse fields of study, including the sciences of play, complex systems, pain, motor control, exercise physiology, and psychology. They show that mainstream formulas for movement health are often seriously off base. The pathway to physical wellness is not about following a recipe, but going on a meaningful adventure.

Issac Asimov noted that scientific truths are usually accessed through unexpected pathways:

> The most exciting phrase to hear in science, the one that heralds new discoveries, is not "Eureka!" (I found it!) but "That's funny ..."

Babies are curious scientists of movement. They are constantly experimenting with different ways to perform important tasks, like how to crawl, drop food off a table, or get a foot into their mouth. They don't know how to do these things, so they need to randomly explore different options until they get an interesting result. When a baby rolls over for the first time, it is often the accidental effect of trying to reach for a toy that is out of grasp. In terms of Asimov's quote, they are probably thinking "hmm that's funny."

Children learn sport skills through play. The impressive moves you see on TV were often learned by improv on the street with other children, rather than formal instruction at an academy. Sports announcers are correct in making the common observation about especially creative plays: "you can't teach that." Even when good technique is taught formally, a more intuitive process of tinkering provides the necessary fine tuning. Practice is often about randomly fiddling with different techniques until things fall into place.

A similar process assists recovery from pain. If your low back starts to hurt, you will start adjusting how to move it, consciously or unconsciously. You might avoid a movement that makes it feel worse, repeat a stretch that makes it feel better, or change your overall level of activity. Playing around with movement is part of a complex healing process that usually resolves the problem in a few weeks. Most back pain is self-limiting, which means it doesn't require a specific treatment to get better.[7] In fact, most treatments for back pain, including exercises to improve core strength and posture, manual therapies like chiropractic and massage, and even many forms of surgery, work no better than "general exercise," which basically means staying physically active in any way that you find meaningful.[8]

None of this means that having a specific plan to improve your physical wellness is a bad idea. Experts in performance or rehab can be extremely helpful, and should be consulted in appropriate circumstances. However, we need to remember they don't have magic pills or simple formulas to cure pain, turn us into elite athletes, or make us "bullet proof." Trainers and therapists often claim the ability to "fix" problems related to movement, in the same way that a mechanic might fix a car. I know because I used to be one of them.

I have been in practice as a manual and movement therapist for more than 12 years. When I got started, I assumed that movement problems could be rather easily "fixed." I was taught that if someone has pain or limited function, you can do objective assessments to find the cause, and then use simple interventions to provide the cure. For example, if your low back feels stiff and appears excessively arched, the cure might be better posture, stronger glutes and abs, or hip stretching. The treatment protocols were like recipes - you follow a series of steps and get the desired result.

These methods sometimes worked, but not consistently. So I sought out advanced trainings with more complicated treatment algorithms. Instead of looking for one of two different causes for pain or dysfunction, I could look for five or six. My assumption was the more I knew, the more accurately I could determine exactly what needed to be done. But I eventually found the opposite – *the more I learned, the more I realized how much more there was to know, and how little of it could be measured or controlled.*

This is a common pattern in complex topics like nutrition, politics, or economics. Before studying, you know nothing, and you know that you know nothing. After you study for a while, you may start to believe you have all the answers, and start annoying friends and family with unwanted advice.[9] But after learning more, and going down various rabbit holes and dead ends, you appreciate the vast complexity of the subject matter. You realize that no matter how much data you acquire, a large degree of uncertainty will remain, and that every particular case is highly individual and contextual. This can lead to some initial despair and confusion, but there is a bright side. You don't need perfect knowledge to resolve complex problems, which paradoxically often have relatively simple solutions.[10]

World class experts in pain will admit the difficulty of answering even seemingly basic questions. What is the cause for low back pain? The best answer is that we usually can't be sure. More than 80% of low back pain is classified "nonspecific," which means that a specific cause for the pain can't be identified.[11] This doesn't mean science hasn't acquired a lot of knowledge about pain. In fact, we know a ton, and I will discuss the most interesting and relevant findings throughout the book. One of the main takeaways is that common musculoskeletal pains often do not require a specific treatment. Most resolve on their own, especially when you have the confidence and willingness to explore different ways to get moving again.[12] Playing with movement is often the simple answer to a complex problem. Similar principles hold for improving sport performance. Top experts in training admit it's very hard to know how work in the gym will transfer to the field of play. The surest path to better function is relatively simple: play the game, making sure to vary its intensity, frequency, and rules.

Although there is much we don't yet know about the human body, one thing is certain: it has an amazing capacity to adapt to the stresses of life and sport by developing a wide range of physical skills and capacities. This book is about helping you explore different ways to play with movement, to develop whatever abilities you want.* Here is a brief overview of its contents:

CHAPTER 1 provides a model of movement health, arguing that it is a multidimensional construct that can only be understood by viewing it from many different perspectives, including structural, physiological, coordinative, psychological, perceptive, sociological, and environmental.

CHAPTER 2 explains why play is an ideal way to build multidimensional movement health and solve complex movement problems. All animals

---

* My first book, *A Guide to Better Movement*, addressed similar topics, but with a very different emphasis, focusing exclusively on the role of the nervous system in movement health. This book is far broader, looking at movement health from a multi-dimensional perspective.

and children develop a wide variety of movement skills and capacities primarily through spontaneous play and not organized practice.

CHAPTER 3 delves further into the nature of complexity by looking at basic concepts from complex systems theory, including variability, non-linearity, feedback loops, self-organization, and attractor states. These concepts provide great insight into how we adapt to stress, coordinate movement, and recover from pain. They also help explain why reductionist methods, which can work medical miracles in certain cases, can be relatively powerless and even counterproductive when used on complex problems.

CHAPTER 4 looks at stress physiology as a way to understand how we adapt to physical and emotional challenges. Chronic stress is a killer, but exercise is a form of stress that is incredibly healthy. What doesn't kill us will make us stronger, but only in the right kind and amount.

CHAPTERS 5-11 examine, in turn, one of the dimensions of movement health discussed in the movement health model:

- fitness
- environment, both social and physical
- musculoskeletal structure
- posture
- mobility
- skill and coordination
- pain

In each chapter, I will discuss the complexity of the subject matter, the many myths on the topic that have arisen due to a reductionist perspective, and some common sense and actionable ways that we can play with movement to improve this particular dimension of movement health. Consistent with the systems-based perspective of the book, each chapter will emphasize the interdependence of the different dimensions. For example, mobility is in many ways about strength, strength requires coordination, coordination is affected by pain, and so forth. Each chapter will give you a different perspective on movement health and new ideas about how to play with movement.

This book will not encumber you with any recipes or specific methods. But it will explain some general principles that apply to any method, and which can help you take control of your movement health in a way that is fun, meaningful, and empowering. Let's get started.

1

MOVEMENT HEALTH

It is more important to know what sort of person has a disease, than to know what sort of disease a person has.
—HIPPOCRATES

All models are wrong but some are useful.
—GEORGE BOX

What does it mean to be a healthy mover? Let's look at some examples. Who is a good model of movement health?

- A person in a wheelchair who competes in marathons.
- A pro basketball player who needs daily medication to deal with chronic pain.
- A yoga master who can fully relax in contorted postures and spends most days in sedentary meditation.
- A powerlifter who can squat 800 pounds, but is so muscular he waddles like a duck.
- An ultra-marathoner who can barely do five push-ups.
- A professional soccer player with chronic fatigue syndrome.

- A fitness model who hates to exercise.
- A hunter gatherer who can live in complete independence.
- A mother of three with unexplained back pain, who is active, happy, and socially engaged.

Of course we cannot objectively rank these people into some kind of hierarchy. There are many different ways to move and feel, and questions about which are best are inherently subjective. But looking at the above examples can get us thinking about the different reasons we value physical wellness. Many different variables seem to matter, and you can have some without the others. Some people value strength, others fitness or skill. Some people just want to feel good while hiking or playing with their kids. Others don't care so much how they feel – their priority is to explore their physical potential, and pain is just part of the journey. The bottom line is that everyone has their own conception of what it means to have movement health.

The traditional definition of health in the medical establishment is simply the absence of disease.[1] Current definitions are more nuanced and expansive,[2] but the old-school attitude lingers. Imagine going to the doctor feeling achy, tired and weak. You get a detailed examination, all the tests come back negative, and he declares that you are perfectly health. This is unsatisfying. A better conception of health would include feeling resilient, happy and capable.[3] But these qualities tend to get ignored by mainstream medicine because they are not objective, and therefore not easily measured like broken bones or infections. The difficulty in defining health is that it is complex. If it was an object, it would be multi-dimensional, with many different sides - musculoskeletal, cognitive, emotional, cardiovascular, etc.

This broader conception of health was incorporated into the highly influential biopsychosocial (BPS) model, developed by George Engel in 1977.[4] The BPS model was intended to improve on the prevailing "biomedical" model, which focused on treating specific diseases, thereby ignoring general wellness. One of the premises of the BPS model is that

A GOOD
QUESTION
TO
ASK

health problems often can't be isolated to a specific part of the body, and that "single-factor thinking" can lead us astray.

Here's an example of how the two methods might differ in their approach to treating shoulder pain associated with a torn rotator cuff. The biomedical model would see the torn rotator cuff as the disease and this would suggest surgery as the cure. The biopsychosocial approach would view the problem from different perspectives, thereby recognizing a broader array of potential solutions. For example, poor coordination might be a contributing factor for the shoulder pain — perhaps the rotator cuff is damaged because it is not properly stabilized in the socket. Maybe muscle weakness is a reason for the poor coordination. Or, maybe the condition of the rotator cuff is not the key problem, because it is quite common, even normal, to have a torn rotator cuff and no pain at all. Pain might arise only in the presence of heightened pain sensitivity, which might be caused by inflammation, lack of activity, poor diet, or insomnia. A psychological perspective would appreciate that musculoskeletal pain is associated with fear of movement and emotional stress. This would suggest treatments based on pain education and stress reduction. Perhaps stress is caused by social factors, such as a 70-hour workweek or recent divorce. Now we have a very large set of potential targets to aim at for pain treatment.

So what is the true cause for the shoulder pain and what is the best solution? There isn't any *one* answer to this question. There are multiple causes for the shoulder pain. This answer can be frustrating if we are determined to pinpoint the exact reason for a problem, or the precise recipe to fix it. But there is a bright side — if a problem has multiple causes, there are more ways to resolve it. Shoulder pain might be successfully treated through surgery, physical therapy, exercise, diet, improved sleep, stress reduction, or just education about the causes for pain. This suggests a treatment approach that is personalized, exploratory, flexible, and, importantly, *does not necessarily require expert assistance.*

We could apply similar reasoning to athletic performance, which always depends on complex interactions between multiple variables:

strength, fitness, motivation, meaning, community, sleep, coordination, training load, stress, injury, personal relationships, diet, etc. Performance might be improved by turning any one of many different dials. Figuring out which ones matter for any particular circumstance is more art than science, and will always require some trial and error.[5]

THE MANY DIMENSIONS OF MOVEMENT HEALTH

If physical wellness is a multidimensional construct, we can only understand it by viewing it from multiple perspectives. If we insist on choosing the one "correct" viewpoint, we are bound to miss something important. With that in mind, I have listed below some examples of different "dimensions" of movement health. Some of these are commonly overrated by the traditional biomedical model, while others tend be neglected. The list below isn't definitive or exhaustive — we could add additional items, subdivide them into different subcategories, or describe them with different terms. The point is to look at movement problems through different lenses, as a way to see a wider range of potential solutions.

Structure

Physical health obviously has a structural dimension. To perform any kind of task, you need some threshold level of muscularity, bone density, and joint integrity. Put simply, you need the right hardware to move well. Football players must be thick and heavily muscled, ballet dancers need hip joints that are free to move easily, and runners need springy Achilles tendons that can handle the stress of repeated pounding.

In our culture, physical structure tends to be overrated. One reason is that we are very concerned with appearances, and structure is quite visible. Another is that structure is easily measured and quantified, and therefore gets a lot of attention from surgeons, chiropractors, and athletic coaches looking to apply scientific principles to movement. Chapter 7 will discuss many common myths related to structure, especially its role in chronic pain. In particular, we will review a large body of research looking at the surprising lack of correlation between pain and common structural issues like bulging discs, torn rotator cuffs and damaged knees. We will also examine evidence calling into question the efficacy of numerous orthopedic surgeries to correct these conditions.

Fitness

Fitness means preparedness to do physical work. It is to some extent "specific," meaning that being fit to perform one kind of task, such as running a marathon, does not guarantee fitness for another one, such as lifting heavy weights. This is why fitness is divided into different sub-categories, such as strength, endurance and mobility.

Although fitness is to some degree specific, there is such a thing as being generally fit. For example, if you can run a seven-minute mile, or perform a bodyweight barbell squat, it's a pretty good guess that you are fit to perform many other tasks. As we'll discuss in Chapter 5, there's a large body of research finding that fitness is correlated with all sorts of positive health outcomes. You can develop well-rounded fitness with a relatively playful approach — one that is fun, favors variety, and avoids repetitive specialization. However, if you want to reach an elite level of fitness in any area, you will need to do some hard work and specialize, and just playing around will probably not get the job done.

Recovery

Fitness requires that you move, but also that you rest after moving. Stress plus recovery equals growth. If you don't fully recover, you can't fully adapt. Nor can you handle chronic stress, which has the potential to severely undermine your health and fitness. This means that a key aspect of building movement health is getting enough sleep, spending quality time with friends and family, eating well, and minimizing sources of emotional stress. The balance between excitement and relaxation is also required for skill development. The optimal learning environment combines elements of intense focus with unstructured exploration. A playful attitude is one that strikes an appropriate balance between challenge and recovery. We will discuss this balance in chapters four and five.

Skill

Movement skill is the ability to efficiently solve movement problems, such as how to lift a bag of groceries, ascend the stairs, or perform a respectable downward-facing dog pose. Some movement skills are more or less essential components of movement health. Postural balance, walking, running, squatting, climbing, reaching, jumping and landing are all fundamental. If you struggle to perform any of these basic actions, your overall movement fluency will be impaired. Other movement skills are highly specific, meaning they are necessary to perform one particular task, and almost nothing else. Playing good pool is a wonderful thing, and one of my favorite activities, but it's probably not making a positive contribution to my basic physical wellness.

In general, fundamental movement skills are easily developed through playful methods, while more complex and specific skills usually require some work. Chapters 9 and 10 address the nature of good movement skills, how we learn them, and whether they matter for health or pain. Some of the major takeaways are that play is an effective way to learn, the game is the best teacher, and simple "corrective" recipes for posture and fundamental movement patterns are significantly overrated.

Perception

Movement skill is almost inseparable from accurate perception about the position of the body in relation to the environment. Thus, learning movement skill is very much about developing perceptual abilities. Further, protective responses such as pain and stress depend on perception: they are activated by the perception of threat, whether or not a real threat exists. These are just a few of the many ways that mind and body are connected, which we will discuss throughout the book, especially in the chapters on stress, movement skill, and pain.

Psychological

Movements have an emotional aspect — they feel good, or bad, and this makes us want to repeat them or avoid them. The feeling that gets our attention most readily is pain. There are many other affective "flavors" associated with movement. Walking, running, or dancing might feel stiff, heavy, awkward, fatiguing or just "wrong." Or they might feel deeply right — revitalizing, powerful, skillful, or expressive.

Athletic performance requires the right mood. To play your best, you need to be aroused and focused, but not too nervous. Play is associated with a psychological state that gets you motivated to move, and to perform well while moving.

Social

Humans are social animals and everything that matters to us — family, friends, jobs, wealth — depends in part on personal relationships. Therefore, movement always has a social dimension, and this is easily overlooked. An athlete's performance depends on interactions with coaches, teammates, competitors and spectators. The most popular forms of exercise — CrossFit, yoga, Zumba, Body Pump, and spin class — get people energized through group dynamics. Social factors can also be powerful inhibitors of movement. The phrase "dance like no one is watching" has a negative corollary — people are often incapable of physically expressing themselves in the presence of other people. Further, many kids learn to hate sports or even physical activity because they receive negative judgments from others about their performance. We all fall into social grooves, and these play a major role in determining how we move.

Environment

[handwritten note: HOW TO STRUCTURE ENVIRONMENT TO PROMOTE MVMT]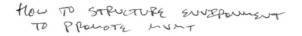

Our movement behavior is affected by the presence of "affordances," features of the environment that "invite" us to move in certain ways. Green fields, hiking trails, playgrounds and dance floors all encourage us to get moving. Other environments tell us to stop moving and sit still: a town with wide streets and no sidewalks; a neighborhood without parks or green spaces; a job that requires constant typing; a living space with couches all pointed at the TV. Many of our current problems with movement health "live" more in the modern environment than the people.

A MODEL FOR MOVEMENT HEALTH

Now that we have looked at various dimensions of physical wellness, let's consider how they relate to each other. Figure 1.1 shows a network of factors that interact in a dynamic way to create a complex whole. Here are several points worth noting.

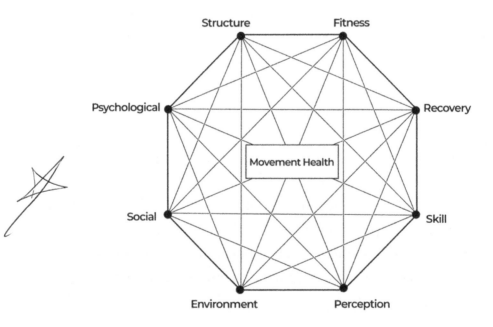

Figure 1.1: Movement health as a complex, multi-dimensional network of relationships between different factors.

First, the different dimensions overlap and do not establish distinct categories. For example, all social events are necessarily psychological events as well. Coordination cannot really be separated from body perception, because one depends on the other. Part of fitness is having a healthy structure. Thus, the different dimensions are not about dividing a complex whole into some neat little boxes, but providing different perspectives to look at it. We could easily add or subtract perspectives, divide them into different subcategories, or label them differently.

Second, the model is not a pyramid, so there is no hierarchical relationship between the different factors. It's a network, where all the relationships are mutually supportive, like strands of a spider web. Thus, there are multiple entry points to improving the overall health of the system. Strength might be improved by working on coordination, or vice versa. This is in contrast to a linear model, which might dictate that coordination must come before strength, or this will increase the risk for injury. Other models actually recommend the opposite — strength should always be the foundation for good function. The reality is that there is no one plan that fits every person and circumstance. Instead, goals can be reached through many different pathways. Better fitness will generally help you move with more coordination. Getting out of pain can make you stronger and vice versa. Running might be improved by beneficial changes in sleep, strength, psychological state, social dynamics, environment, fitness, or coordination.

Third, placing too much priority on one particular aspect of physical wellness might cause a general imbalance. If you want to have elite endurance, you will need to compromise on other aspects of your movement health. Conversely, correcting a major deficiency in one area might bring general benefits. For someone who is very physically weak, resistance training might be a game changer. Some of the dimensions of movement health tend to get systematically ignored by the mainstream, while others get overemphasized. In general, most of our attention tends toward objectively measurable and conspicuously visible factors like structure or fitness. And we ignore the more subjective concepts related to psychology and perception. Throughout the book, you will see this pattern appear repeatedly, especially in relation to the way chronic pain is commonly treated. A related theme is that play is a good way to restore emphasis to some of the overlooked areas and promote multi-dimensional movement health.

One last thing to remember about the model: it's just a model! It does not purport to be a full representation of everything we need to know about movement health. In fact, no model can meet this criterion — some form of simplification is always required. With this in mind, it has been said that all models are wrong but some are useful. As I see it, the above model is useful to the extent that it reminds us that movement problems are usually complex and need to be considered from many different angles. If you are struggling with one approach, use another.

2

PLAY

*I played everything. I played soccer, lacrosse,
track and field, and hockey.*
—WAYNE GRETZSKY

*I tell you, we are here on Earth to fart around,
and don't let anybody tell you different.*
—KURT VONNEGUT

Why do animals play? Imagine two cheetah cubs wrestling as their mother tries to nap. Every once in a while, they crash into her face and wake her up. She's a good sport though, tolerating the foolishness for a bit, before batting them away and getting some more rest. Later that day, the cubs are playing again, chasing each other, and eventually they almost get lost. Mom retrieves them, so they don't get eaten by hyenas. That night, Mom is stalking some gazelles for dinner (which the cubs need to replenish the energy they spent earlier in the day annoying Mom). As Mom is getting ready to strike, the cubs are roughhousing, eventually blundering out into the open, scaring away their dinner.

How would an animal scientist look at this seemingly wasteful behavior? When viewed from an evolutionary perspective, play may appear to be a paradox, because it has some very obvious costs and no obvious benefits. In addition to annoying Mom, it consumes energy, exposes the cubs to increased risk of predation and injury, and diverts attention from other important activities, such as hunting. Why would animals evolve an instinct to engage in an activity with these liabilities? According to the logic of natural selection, the answer is that it must have some benefits that exceed the costs.[1] Otherwise, animals with a less playful nature would have outcompeted the playful ones, and we know that didn't happen. So what is the benefit of play?

One answer is that play helps animals build resilient bodies, develop physical fitness, learn movement and social skills, and become more adaptable and creative in general.[2] All intelligent animals play, and the more intelligent the animal, the more it plays. Humans are the smartest, most adaptable animals, and play the most. And they do the most playing at times of life when they need to do the most learning and developing. Therefore, play must somehow be good at helping the body and mind adapt to the demands of the world, especially when those demands are variable and unexpected.

From this perspective, the cheetah cubs play because it's an effective form of "training" for the hard job of being an adult cheetah. Their play is a kind practice of some of the skills they will use in the hunt — stalking, chasing, pouncing, biting, wrestling. And it also develops a general ability to respond creatively to a broad range of unexpected challenges.

But is this playing around really the best way to get that training done? Here's an interesting question: Would the cheetahs be better prepared for their adult lives as badass hunters and stars of nature shows if they went through a process that was more like how modern humans train to be competitive athletes? What if they "worked" at movement instead of playing?

The training process could start with some assessments. Sport scientists could analyze the physical characteristics of the best cheetah hunters to find the optimal levels of speed, strength, agility and endurance. Then they could assess the cheetah trainees to find areas where improvement is needed. For example, one cub might have excellent speed but poor endurance. Another lacks agility, or leg strength, or range of motion. To correct deficiencies, specific drills could be devised: One-hundred-meter sprint repeats for speed endurance; running around cones for agility; repeated jumps for explosive power; stretching to improve range of motion. Of course the cheetahs don't really want to do these things, so they need to be constantly bribed with treats (Wildebeest jerky) after each rep.

The efficiency of the training process could be maximized with a planned schedule of training blocks. The first six months would develop basic movement patterns, then they would add aerobic fitness, and after that a strength phase, then plyometrics and power development. With all this training, the cubs have less time for play and social life, which makes them a bit stressed and ornery. So the scientists make sure the cubs get adequate sleep and nutrition, and monitor their cortisol levels and other stress markers to prevent over training. Is this program likely to produce better hunters than the all-natural, organic version?

Silly question of course, but it serves to distinguish a play-based approach from one that is work-based, involving precise measurements of objective variables like weights, times, and distances, and where discipline is required to complete tasks that are unpleasant and intrinsically meaningless. Which program is better? Should we get out of the gym and start running around like cavemen? Of course we don't need to choose — we can incorporate elements of work and play into our exercise programs, and that is actually what I recommend in this book. But it's good to be aware of the strengths and weaknesses of either approach.

On the one hand, we shouldn't be too romantic about the value of play. The "naturalistic fallacy" is the mistaken idea that whatever is "natural" is good, and whatever is "unnatural" is toxic. This is obviously not true — it is a very natural thing for cheetah cubs to sometimes get eaten by hyenas, or for playful human kids to fall out of trees and break their legs. It is also unnatural for humans to do resistance training on machines in modern gyms, and science shows this can be healthy on multiple levels. Point in favor of working out in safe air-conditioned gyms without hyenas roaming around.

On the other hand, there is such a thing as an "evolutionary mismatch," which occurs when an animal is exposed to an environment that is radically different from the one in which it evolved.[3] Zoo animals often become sick or stressed in unnatural conditions. The modern world is in some ways a zoo for humans, and may be contributing to "diseases of civilization." Obesity, diabetes and heart disease are almost non-existent in hunter-gatherer cultures. Humans are not well adapted to regulate their fitness and weight in environments where Twinkies and frozen pizzas can be purchased at the very low metabolic cost of driving to the nearest 7-Eleven.

We should also be mindful of Orgel's second law of biology, which is that "evolution is cleverer than you are." This means the "designs" that emerge from millions of years of natural selection, including behavioral instincts, are very good solutions to whatever problems they evolved to solve, and therefore our attempts to improve on them are likely to fail. If evolution designed animals to play as a means to train them up to be heathy and functional movers, we would be wise to think twice before concluding we have a better way to go about it. Play is the best tool for developing movement health that natural selection has come up with. That should make us curious about how incorporating more play into our exercise programs might be beneficial.

PLAY AND DEVELOPMENT

Like cheetahs, humans develop the fundamental skills and fitness they need to be healthy movers through self-directed play. Even in modern societies, where unstructured free time is in increasingly short supply, children usually gain a basic level of general movement competency and fitness by the time they are seven, without any instruction. Here's a quick list of functions the vast majority of elementary school kids can perform with ease.

- Retaining postural control and balance in multiple static and dynamic conditions: sitting, standing, squatting, lunging, walking, running.
- Full range of motion reaching with the arms at multiple angles, in coordination with movements of the trunk.
- Sitting comfortably for extended periods in multiple positions: deep squat, kneeling, half-kneeling, cross-legged, extended legs, etc.
- Rolling back and forth from multiple positions: supine, prone, sitting, and standing.
- Lowering to the ground in multiple ways: squatting, lunging, half-kneeling, etc.
- Various forms of locomotion: crawling, walking, running, sprinting, skipping, shuffling.
- Climbing, hanging, swinging and brachiating from overhead supports.
- Jumping onto elevated surfaces, and landing jumps from elevated surfaces, from standing or on the run.
- Moving with agility, i.e. quickly changing directions to avoid or pursue objects or people.

We take many of the above skills for granted, but we shouldn't. Many experts in physical therapy or athletic training will routinely assess their clients' ability to perform these basic functions (e.g., squatting or overhead reaching), and find they are lacking. Interestingly, these same experts often consider children to be ideal models of correct movement. And yet children learn to do these things without assessments or corrections from experts. There are thousands of YouTube videos on how to squat, but children haven't watched any of them.

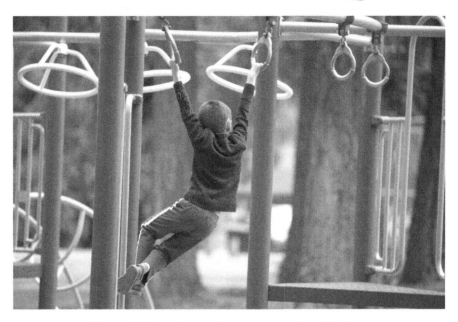

Figure 2.1: A primate demonstrates brachiation.

Play has been held in high esteem by educational theorists for hundreds of years. Philosophers from Rousseau to John Dewey have argued that children learn best when their natural interests are nurtured instead of suppressed.[4] The word kindergarten literally means "garden for children," and reflects the idea that child development is grown not engineered.

Hunter-gatherer children generally don't receive formal education, but they learn a tremendous volume of information and skills before becoming productive adult members of the tribe. Through play and imitation, they learn botany, animal behavior, tool construction, food preparation, hunting technique, and many other things.[5] In the modern world, parents will notice how frighteningly easy it is for kids to learn how to use phones, iPads and computers, without any parental help, and often in the face of significant discouragement. My seven-year-old daughter has better computer literacy than my mother, even though Mom has taken classes. My daughter's learning methods are less formal. She picks up the phone (steals it actually) and then plays around with it, exploring different ways to use it, making plenty of mistakes, and eventually figuring out how to get a rewarding result. Unlike Mom, she enjoys what she is doing, and is led by her curiosity. Most of her know-how is unconscious — she has no explicit knowledge about how to get things done, she just knows how to do them. Mom worries about making mistakes, overanalyzes, and doesn't learn anything unless she writes it down, references later, and eventually memorizes it.

An amazing example of learning through exploration is the "hole in the wall experiment."[6] An Indian physicist placed a computer with internet access into a concrete wall in one of the poorest slums of India. The computer attracted attention from street kids aged 6-12 who had never seen such an object before. Within days, and with no instruction, the kids were playing games and surfing the internet. Would they have learned as quickly if they were compelled to work at it in a structured classroom?

Sport provides another example of play-based learning. In games requiring high levels of technical skill, such as basketball and soccer, the most gifted athletes often emerge from unstructured environments.[7] Brazilian soccer players and American basketball players often learn their skills in pick-up games, and are renowned for their innovation, technical skill, and ability to improvise.[8] The best baseball players in the world currently come from the Dominican Republic. Many of them got their start using broomsticks to hit bottle caps.[9]

Some of the all-time greats, including Wayne Gretzky, Ronaldhino, and Johan Cruyff, specifically credit play and pure love of the game as the basis for their success. They express concern that overly regimented training methods, including early sport specialization, are counterproductive. Research supports this belief and suggests that long-term athletic development is best achieved by letting kids play as many different sports as they want until at least the early teens, saving specialization for later.[10] Here's a quote from Wayne Gretzky, highly regarded as the best hockey player of all time, talking about his multi-sport background:

> I was absolutely ecstatic to see the end of the hockey season. One of the worst things to happen to the game, in my opinion, has been year-round hockey and, in particular, summer hockey. All it does for kids, as far as I can tell, is keep them out of sports they should be doing in warmer weather... All the good hockey players seemed to play lacrosse in those days and every one of them learned something from the game to carry over to the other — things athletes can only learn by mixing up games they play when they are young.

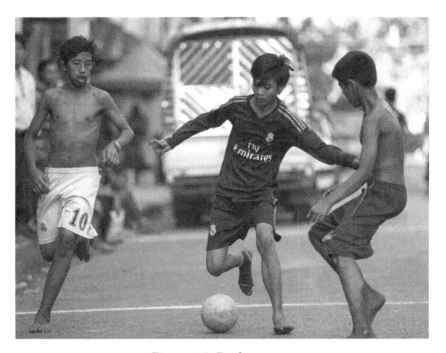

Figure 2.2: Real soccer.

None of this means that play is the only way to learn. Many skills will not simply emerge naturally during unstructured exploration, and they will take some hard work to master. This is particularly true in highly technical sports like golf or gymnastics. But no matter how advanced you get, play remains a source of creativity and growth.

PLAY DEFINED

We know play when we see it in the most obvious cases like kids chasing each other on a playground, or puppies wrestling. But for adults, the line between work and play is not always clear. For example, consider a man running on a treadmill. Sounds like work. What if he is running on a trail in a beautiful environment? That might be enjoyable. Two men kicking around a soccer ball might be playing. What if they are professionals getting ready for a game? Is that work? What if they are laughing and showing off with juggling tricks? Are highly competitive ten-year-old gymnasts playing as they repeat back flips? What about a tai chi student repeating a form he has done a thousand times, but in a state of blissed-out concentration?

There has been a good deal of scientific inquiry into play behavior in animals and children, and its effects on cognitive and physical health.[11] There is also psychological research concerning the nature and benefits of "flow" states, and the effects of different kinds of motivation on exercise adherence. None of these sources define play in exactly the same way, or with bright line definitions, but certain themes and common factors emerge. Here are some of the ways that play is distinct from work.

PLAY IS INTRINSICALLY MOTIVATING

John Dewey said that "playful activities are enjoyable in their own execution without reference to ulterior purpose."[12] Mark Twain put it more simply: "Work consists of whatever a body is obliged to do. Play consists of whatever a body is not obliged to do." Experts in animal behavior consider an activity to be play when it doesn't serve any obvious short-term goal related to survival or reproduction.[13] When you see two animals chasing each other around, and one is not trying to eat or mate with the other one, they are probably playing. Play isn't serving some larger purpose, it's an end in itself.

This definition is a bit harder to apply to humans. A man running on a beach might find the activity enjoyable, but he might have other motivations. Running helps him lose weight, maintains his heart health, and gets him ready to compete in an upcoming 5K. If it weren't for these incentives, he might prefer a walk to a run. After all, running is hard, and he must expend at least some degree of willpower to continue. Does a Labrador retriever need willpower to chase a ball? No, that is exactly what it wants to do. Some humans are just as motivated to move as a dog chasing a ball. Many dancers, surfers, skiers, and golfers would rather dance, surf, ski and golf than almost anything else, and would happily sacrifice their wealth and social status to do so. For them, the activity is definitely an end in itself.

What about activities that we are motivated to do, but aren't necessarily "fun"? Running or weightlifting requires serious effort, and causes some degree of suffering. And yet, many people feel a deep need to do these activities almost every day, because they are part of a physical practice that feels meaningful. The search for meaning is probably a stronger motivator and contributor to well-being than the search for pleasure. Good feelings are of course a wonderful thing, but the pursuit of happiness presents a paradox — seeking it out tends to make it harder to achieve. Further, a positive mood without a sense of meaning may feel shallow.[14] As applied to physical activity, this explains why many people would choose a grueling run over playing Twister or hopscotch.

This highlights an important point. **Play is not about doing things that are immature, frivolous, or trivial. It is about getting absorbed in an activity that is intrinsically motivating.** When kids are playing at drawing a picture, assembling a tower of blocks, or learning to crawl, they are making serious efforts to accomplish important goals. This process can certainly be fun, but it is not all "fun and games."

The psychologist Mihaly Csikszentmihalyi coined the term "flow" to refer to deeply rewarding and meaningful experiences that occur when people are completely absorbed in an activity that requires skill and concentration to perform well.[15] One of its qualities is the feeling that effective actions are occurring automatically, spontaneously, or effortlessly, without the need for excessive self-consciousness or will-power. The Buddhist philosopher Alan Watts referred to this state as being "the real secret of life — to be completely engaged with what you are doing in the here and now. And instead of calling it work, realize it is play."

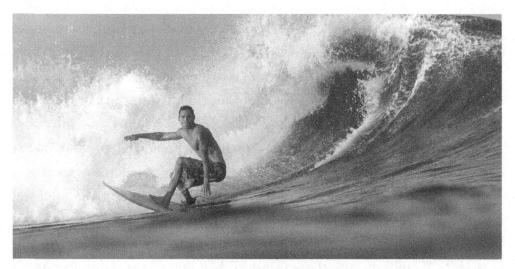

Figure 2.3: Flow.

The opposite end of the spectrum from play/flow is work/drudgery — exercise that feels miserable, requires major resources of willpower and conscious control to complete, and is only done for some extrinsic benefit. Far from being the first thing you want to do, it might even be the last. People stairmastering in the gym often hate the experience, but are willing to endure it to lose weight, get a six pack, improve their health, and maybe even watch TV at the same time. If they could get these benefits from a pill, they would stop stairmastering immediately and never do it again. This is completely different from an avid runner or weightlifter, who might be doing a similar kind of physical work, and is in some sense feeling as much pain, but *wants* to engage in the activity, and even finds it an essential part of their mental health.

YES!   *FLOW*

Exercise that is unpleasant and meaningless might burn the exact same calories as exercise that creates a state of flow. But the psychology is very different, and this has important consequences. One is the decreased likelihood of showing up to do more exercise tomorrow, next week, or next year. Research shows that people who exercise because they enjoy it, or because it gives them a personal sense of mastery, are more likely to adhere to their fitness plans than people who are motivated by "body reasons" like looking better in selfies or swimsuits.[16] Further, adherence is higher when exercise provides an immediate sense of gratification, compared to a distant reward in the future.[17]

Second, boring workouts do not have the same physical effects as identical activities that are enjoyable. Emotional states affect the body through the endocrine, autonomic and nervous systems. We all know that too much worrying can cause a headache, ulcer, or even heart attack. Stress is a major cause of disease, and a big predictor of pain and injury as well. Psychology is inseparable from physiology. Therefore, an enjoyable five-mile run done in 40 minutes will promote movement health better than the same exact run that is boring, meaningless and stressful. We will discuss these mind-body connections in greater detail in chapters four and eleven.

& SUPPORTS STRESS RECOVERY

PLAY IS NOT TOO STRESSFUL

Animals and babies generally stop playing when they are sick or stressed out.[18] If you haven't eaten for several days, this isn't a good time for some major roughhousing or capture the flag. Play, almost by definition, never compromises the recovery dimension of movement health.

So animals and kids have the good sense to avoid optional physical activities when they need to rest. But competitive adult humans can get carried away. They love to run, dance, or do CrossFit so much that they may continue with these activities even when they are highly stressful. Professional athletes get paid to play hurt, but the rest of us do not, so play should probably be considered work when it becomes more than moderately painful.

Another interesting distinction is between play and contest.[19] Experts in animal behavior note major differences between play fighting, which is basically about having fun, and ritualized fighting, whose purpose is to establish a dominance hierarchy that will determine access to resources, such as mating partners or territory. Big difference!

In play fighting, the stronger animal will let the weaker one "win" from time to time, by lying on its back, or otherwise handicapping itself. Because if it doesn't, the weaker one will just get bored and find someone to play with who isn't a bully. But a contest for resources is not about having fun or making sure everyone gets a trophy. It is a hard-core zero-sum game with a winner and a loser, and very real consequences. The animals may not fight to the death, but they fight hard enough to determine who will be dead if things keep going. The loser goes home with diminished prospects for life and lower levels of testosterone. The winner claims the prize of better hunting territory or mating opportunities.[20]

In humans, the line between play and contest is sometimes blurred. All sports involve at least some element of contest, because there is some degree of social status at stake. But that doesn't mean there's no element of play involved. Competitive sports are usually enjoyable, especially when played with good sportsmanship. Of course, sport may sometimes cross the line into something that is not very fun at all. Most people have a strong intuitive sense of when a friendly game of pick-up basketball degenerates into something that is far less healthy. If losing makes you feel ashamed, depressed or stressed, you are probably not playing anymore.

PLAY IS EXPLORATORY

Play has a curious attitude and favors exploration over following a map. Babies don't need coaching in how to move, they just figure things out on their own. When they are learning to roll over, no one is telling them to activate their core or fire their glutes. (Except in exclusive neighbor-hoods in San Francisco.) Instead, they experiment with different move-ment strategies almost at random, most of which fail miserably. The developmental psychologist Esther Thelen describes the process:

> Young mammals—including children—spend a lot of time in behavior with no apparent goal. They move, they jiggle, they run around, they bounce things and throw them, and gener-ally abuse them in ways that seem, to mature minds, to have no good use. However, this behavior, commonly called play, is essential to building inventive forms of intelligence that are open to new solutions.[21]

According to Thelen, babies learn through exploration of different options, and then repetition of what works. After some repetitions, there needs to be further experimentation to make sure they haven't settled on a suboptimal solution. For example, babies' first attempts at crawling might move them forward in a worm-like manner, which is not very efficient. So they will continue to explore different solutions, and eventually discover contralateral crawling and walking. Play scien-tist Patrick Bateson believes that play evolved as a way to help animals avoid "false endpoints" — solutions that are workable but not opti-mal.[22] This idea is sometimes explained with the metaphor of a climber searching a landscape for the highest peak, without a full view of the area. If your strategy is to simply keep moving upward, you will soon reach a local peak. But to find the global peak, you need to occasion-ally descend, walk through some valleys, and explore new areas.

PLAY IS CREATIVE

Sport cultures that value a playful approach often produce athletes who are especially creative. Brazil is known for a style of soccer that is not only effective, but aesthetically pleasing. Pele called soccer the "beautiful game," and it is learned in unstructured play, not formal competition.

Highly creative people, like Mozart, Einstein, and Picasso, acknowledge that play is essential for productivity. Here's an excellent line about the value of exploration in reaching distant goals, from Bill Watterson, the creator of the *Calvin and Hobbes* comics: "The truth is, most of us discover where we are headed when we arrive." The physicist Richard Feynman arrived at a Nobel prize by following a seemingly useless train of thought about the wobbling movements of a dinner plate:

> It was effortless. It was easy to play with these things. It was like uncorking a bottle: Everything flowed out effortlessly. I almost tried to resist it![23]

Feynman's state of mind sounds a lot like the flow state described by Csikszentmihalyi: a feeling of effortless mastery, uncontrolled by conscious planning. Athletes and dancers report similar feelings when exploring all the different way their bodies can move. Their curiosity often leads to the development of seemingly impractical skills. For example, soccer players juggle balls on their shoulders and balance them on their heads. Basketball players spin balls on their fingers, and dribble two balls at once. Golfers can strike perfect drives out of mid-air after dropping the ball from their hand. These tricks have no practical value, but the attitude which led to their discovery is part of what allowed them to master their sport.

PLAY IS TINKERING

Play is sometimes used as a synonym for tinkering. It means trying to resolve a problem by fiddling around with different variables in a semi-random manner. This is in contrast to a more workmanlike strategy, which relies on precise planning. Tinkering is different — you solve a problem just by messing around, and things tend to sort themselves out of their own accord. You probably won't even know how you got the result.

Consider a pro baseball player whose swing feels off. He might go to the batting cage and start playing around with different grips, swing paths, or ways to focus his attention. There is no real plan, just messing around with different possibilities, and then waiting for things to fall back into place. This is similar to how you might try to fix a stalled computer: Close down some apps; turn the computer on and off; change some settings. After some futzing around, the problem resolves.

The same thing happens with pain. If your shoulder starts to hurt while doing a push-up, the first thing you will do is start making some adjustments to your form. This happens spontaneously and unconsciously. You might slow your speed, move your hands a little bit further apart, or adjust your trunk angle. After a few repetitions of playing around, the shoulder now feels comfortable. Now imagine you are in a class with an instructor telling you exactly how you need to be moving, prescribing the "correct" hand placement, technique, sets and reps. Or worse yet, telling you that you need to stop moving right away and go to the doc. This might inhibit the natural tinkering process that would have solved the problem.

PLAY INVOLVES RISK

Play is a way to test the efficiency of different movements, and also their safety.[24] In fact, playful behaviors often involve some element of risk. When cheetah cubs play, they learn how fast they can run without falling, how hard they can fight without getting hurt, and how much they can bother Mom before she gets mad. Human kids do the same thing. They learn where the lines are by crossing them repeatedly. There's risk in stepping too far, but also risk in not stepping far enough, and failing to discover the limits of potential. As we age, we start with games that are very safe, and then progress to games with more risk. Many people graduate to doing things that are truly stupid. If they survive, they learn some very valuable lessons (hopefully).

But in the beginning, playful exploration presents little risk. When babies are learning to roll over and crawl, there is no way to get hurt if something goes wrong. Without fear of injury, it's easy to engage in many trials and many errors, and to learn a ton about how to get coordinated.* But they are learning nothing about how to protect themselves. As soon as babies stand up and start walking, their education in the potential risks of movement begins.

Toddlers taking their first steps will fall many times a day. This is unlikely to cause injury because they are close to the ground and have a nice layer of protective fat over their butts. But falling creates nociception, which is the sensory signaling that can result in pain. This puts the nervous system to work in reading evidence about physical threat and deciding whether pain is necessary for protection. Has the butt been injured? Is this a dangerous situation?

There are other important questions raised by falling. Is backward better than forward? Is it a good idea to cry to get Mom's attention? Should we give up on walking for now and return to crawling? Confronting these questions is a form of training in weighing the risks and rewards of various kinds of movement.

As kids get older, they start to play with movements that can cause minor injuries. Jumping off couches or benches, running on sidewalks, or going down slides will frequently bruise knees and scrape hands. Each fall is a learning opportunity — did I get injured, how long will it hurt, will I need a band-aid? If I cry enough, will I get ice cream?

Kids who fall after running often don't know exactly what to think or feel. They were running along without a care in the world, and now they are face down in the dirt. They usually look around for the face of a parent. If Mom is looking panicked and sprinting over, the kid will probably start crying. And if Mom plays it cool, gives a bit of a shrug and

---

* In my previous book, *A Guide to Better Movement*, I offered a series of movement lessons, based on the Feldenkrais Method, that resemble the ground-based explorations of infants. When you're on the floor, it's easier to play with movement, because risk is reduced to a minimum.

smile, the kid usually gets back up and continues to play. Pain always has a social dimension, and kids start learning about it through play.

After getting some significant experience with scraped knees and bruised elbows, kids will start to refine their movement strategies related to self-protection. Some will become cautious, avoiding climbing, contact sports and roughhousing. Better safe than sorry. Other kids take the opposite path: no guts, no glory. They make several trips to the ER before their 6th birthday, but are rewarded by superior skills in skateboarding.

I recently did some soccer coaching for eight-year-old girls, most of them novices. I watched something interesting happen on at least five occasions. A girl got hit with the ball unexpectedly in the thigh, or trunk, or arm. They would look startled, confused, and then start crying about 10 seconds later. They would leave the game, settle down, and then return to the game feeling fine. I think what happened was that they experienced a completely novel and surprising feeling and didn't know what it meant. Eventually they learned that it was not really a problem — the body is pretty tolerant to getting smacked with a soccer ball, and this isn't something that should cause pain.

As kids (especially boys) approach the teenage years, they may start playing with some seriously risky stuff, like fighting, extreme skiing, and football. Some of these "games" may be more in the nature of contests intended to establish dominance hierarchies. Either way, there are important lessons for the players. First, there are many occasions to differentiate between minor and more serious injuries, and this can increase body awareness and refine a sense of threat perception. Scrapes and bruises are very different from sprains and breaks. The former should be pretty much ignored, and the latter requires a trip to the doc. With this sense of perspective in place, minor injuries become more tolerable, and may not even be noticed. Another lesson from risky activities relates to fear management. For example, proper skiing technique (much like asking someone for a date) requires that you lean forward with confidence. You may fall flat on your face, but you need to forget about that for the time being. In many situations, worrying about a bad outcome will make it more likely. Fear is the enemy, and playing with risk is a way to learn to master it. Further, handling a risky situation builds confidence, and a sense of self-efficacy. As we will see later in the book, these qualities are protective against chronic pain and disability.

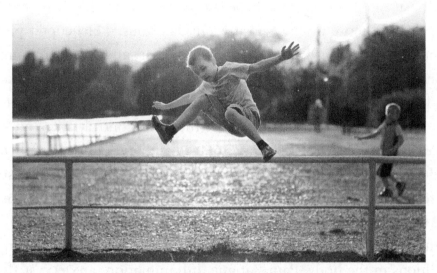

Figure 2.4: Learning about threat.

Peter Gray argues that young mammals have an instinct to "dose" themselves with risky situations as a way to inoculate themselves against the disease of anxiety:

> In their motor play and rough-and-tumble play, juvenile mammals appear to put themselves deliberately into awkward, moderately frightening situations. . . . When they leap, for example, they twist and turn in ways that make it difficult to land. They seem to be dosing themselves with moderate degrees of fear, as if deliberately learning how to deal with both the physical and emotional challenges of the moderately dangerous conditions they generate.[25]

Kids have less chance to do this in the modern world. Gone are the days when parents let kids play unsupervised for hours at a time near trees, fields, streets, or large groups of multi-age kids. These activities are now considered dangerous unless parents are constantly supervising, monitoring, encouraging, discouraging, coaching, hydrating, child-proofing and doing almost everything short of bubble-wrapping their kids. If the parents weren't there, heaven forbid that a child might fall down, get hurt, be exposed to germs, or suffer a temporary drop in self-esteem. Many experts believe this approach actually makes kids less safe, and more fragile, sensitive and anxious.[26] Helicopter parenting pushes kids toward safe spaces like couches, and away from uncontrolled spaces where they might actually engage in some playful activities like climbing a tree, riding a bike or even playing a game of tag. This prevents them for learning that they can control risk, and some argue this is a cause for rising rates of teen anxiety.[27] It is certainly not a good idea to be reckless and irresponsible, but it can be just as destructive to fear and avoid movement that makes you healthy and robust.

All the above points have implications for adults. As I will discuss in later chapters, perception of threat is at the root of many undesirable conditions in the body. Pain, fatigue, inflammation, anxiety, stiffness, and weakness are all caused, at least in part, by the unconscious perception that the body is weak, under attack, incapable, broken, fragile, damaged, vulnerable to threats. Playing with risky movement is one way to build a self-image that is far more robust, strong and capable. So is disregarding the well-intended but counterproductive advice of many overprotective experts who would seek to prevent us from sitting, standing, running, or drawing even a single breath without the "correct" form.

CAN HUMANS PLAY LIKE CHEETAHS?

Now that we have discussed the difference between play and work in the context of human physical activity, let's return to our silly cheetah hypothetical. Should they be working more and playing less? I think we can be pretty sure the cheetahs should stick to their current program.

They don't need to be told how to move or what to do. If they follow their natural instincts related to movement, socializing, and food acquisition, they will enjoy excellent movement health. Is the same thing true for humans?

It depends. We need to distinguish between humans living in a modern world versus the kind of world where we evolved. Hunter-gatherers living a "natural" lifestyle almost uniformly enjoy excellent movement health, and they don't even have a word for exercise.[28] Movement is life. Kids play all day outside because there's no inside. Adults engage in some play, and must also work to get food, which means walking, climbing, running, sprinting, digging, and throwing. If things go well, they carry heavy loads back to camp. When they get back, they spend hours sitting on the ground, often in deep squats. They might also do some skillful manual work with tools, food preparation, clothing and shelters. Later they may do some dancing. A hard day of work will be followed by one with far more rest and recovery. All the physical activity is socially and psychologically meaningful. Presumably these movements provide hunter-gatherers with a diet of movements that is every bit as nutritious and sustaining for humans as the cheetah's movements are for it. None of these healthful outcomes require a plan — they just tend to happen when humans are in the right environment.

But here's the problem: In the modern world, following our instincts and doing what comes "naturally" doesn't work as well. Kids who follow their play instinct might end up spending more time with video games than tree climbing. Adults who want to provide for the family will drive to the office, not walk to the hunt. And relaxing at home means sitting on the couch and not the floor. Just following your bliss and exploring what seems interesting might not get you moving very much. Thus, the reality of our modern life is that most of us will need to work at physical activity to some extent — use discipline, conscious planning, and willpower to get moving. But this doesn't mean we need to forget about the advantages associated with moving in a way that is enjoyable and meaningful. Even in the modern world, a great many people find physical activities that they love to do, and which keep them very healthy. In fact, the modern world offers a distinct benefit in this regard — we have so many choices. Most people have ready access to physical or virtual spaces that can assist them in playing with any physical activity you can imagine — dance, capoeira, skateboarding, yoga, kettlebells … fire-eating. Hopefully the remainder of this book will provide some inspiration to explore these options (probably skip the fire-eating) and find what works for you.

3

COMPLEXITY

The body is a big sagacity, a plurality with one sense,
a war and a peace, a flock and a shepherd.
~FRIEDRICH NIETZSCHE

I am large, I contain multitudes.
—WALT WHITMAN

The first two chapters argued that developing movement health is a complex problem, and that play is a key tool for solving it. In this chapter we take a closer look at the meaning of complexity, and the nature of complex adaptive systems like the human body. This will help us understand how the body adapts to stress, develops fitness, and learns movement skills. It will also make it easier to spot myths that derive from single-factor thinking or analogizing the body to a machine.

Complexity science provides a fascinating lens through which to view the world. If you are not already familiar with the subject matter, learning more will change the way you look at your body, and almost everything else. Some of the ideas are common sense and intuitive, and others are mind-boggling and abstract. When Stephen Hawking was asked what ideas would best advance our understanding of the future world, he predicted that "the next century will be the century of complexity." I think his prediction will hold true in regard to the study of human health and fitness, and many other fields as well.

Complexity science arose in the mid-twentieth century as a response to the perceived limitations of reductionist thinking in understanding economies, social organizations, weather systems, and living things.* Reductionism means trying to understand a large system by "reducing" it to a collection of smaller parts, and then analyzing them separately. For example, we can get a better understanding of cars, human bodies, cells, and atoms by thinking in terms of their different components. This "divide and conquer" strategy is responsible for almost every amazing accomplishment in the history of science, especially physics, chemistry, engineering, and medicine. So there is nothing fallacious about reductionist thinking, or dividing wholes into parts. However, this strategy may be less useful as applied to a complex system for several reasons.

First, it's not easy to divide complex wholes into parts, because their boundaries are fuzzy. As we saw in chapter one, health can't be reduced to discrete categories without making some arbitrary distinctions. The parts of a machine are discrete and easily separated, but body parts literally bleed into one another. Everything is connected in a very messy way, and when you separate them, something important (e.g. life) is lost. In a complex system, the whole is always greater than the sum of its parts.

Another challenge with complex systems is that they may have too many parts (or interactions between them) to measure. This can be a major problem if small gaps in knowledge lead to large prediction errors. This is common in stock markets, weather systems, or political elections, where there is always major uncertainty about future events. If you ask ten experts for long-term predictions in these areas,

* There are many different sciences and theoretical models that study complexity, including systems theory, complex systems theory, dynamic systems theory, chaos theory, and others. They have differences in terminology and application, but there are many ideas in common. The concepts presented in this chapter are relatively simple, and can be found in many of the different models.

you might get ten different answers, and many would not outperform common sense or a coin flip.[1] A similar confusion can be seen with low back pain — many of my clients have received more than five different diagnoses and prescriptions from different experts. The lesson is that with complex problems, more data does not necessarily lead to better understanding. Looking too closely at the details can cause you to miss the big picture.

Complexity science tries to identify big picture patterns that are invisible from a reductionist perspective. This is done by turning attention away from the specific parts in a system, and towards the patterns of interaction between them. This strategy has discovered that systems made from completely different parts might obey similar rules. For example, the body's response to an emergency has a similar dynamic to a stock market crash or cattle stampede — each involve a positive feedback loop. Fractal geometry has noted similarities between the branching patterns of trees, rivers and blood vessels. The behavior of fish in a school is not unlike voters in a democracy, or neurons in a brain.[2] Tuning into these kinds of patterns can help us to see the logic of living things. It is not a substitute for reductionism, but a different lens for problem-solving.

The need for a different perspective has been noted in the context of medical treatment for complex conditions like chronic pain, obesity, diabetes, anxiety, depression or autoimmune disease.[3] Although reductionist thinking is responsible for medical miracles in cases where there is a single problem (e.g. a broken bone or infection), progress has been slow in the treatment of health problems that are multi-factorial. Andrew Ahn and colleagues argue that the reductionist mindset can lead to mechanical thinking:

> When the human body is viewed as a collection of components, the natural inclination of medicine is to **isolate the single factor** that is most responsible for the observed behavior. **Much like a mechanic who repairs a broken car by locating**

the defective part, physicians typically treat disease by identifying that isolatable abnormality.[4]

The tendency to think of bodies like machines has also been noted by Paul Plsek and Trisha Greenhalgh:

> Newton's "clockwork universe," in which big problems can be broken down into smaller ones, analysed, and solved by rational deduction, has strongly influenced the practice of medicine. . . . **But the machine metaphor lets us down badly** when no part of the equation is constant, independent, or predictable. The new science of complex adaptive systems may provide new metaphors that can help us to deal with these issues better.[5]

Here's an example of how the machine metaphor is misleading as applied to human bodies. Proper functioning of a machine requires that all its parts move in a way that is regular and repetitive. If they don't, this is a dysfunction that needs to be fixed. But human bodies benefit from constant change and even minor chaos in the way the different parts interact.[6] This inherent variability is not a weakness, but a source of strength, intelligence and adaptability. There are many other basic concepts from complexity science that are relevant to physical health, including emergence, self-organization, non-linearity, attractor states, and constraints. In this chapter we will look at each.

EMERGENCE

A defining quality of a complex system is the presence of "emergent" properties, which are collective behaviors by the whole system that cannot be found at the level of the parts. Put simply, emergence is when the whole is *way* more than the sum of its parts, in a way that is surprising.[7] If you only observed fish in isolation, you would be very surprised to see what happens when they get together in a large group. They move as a whole unit in organized patterns, even though no fish intends them. In a human brain, intelligence somehow emerges from the interactions of billions of neurons, none of which are individually smarter than a bacterium.

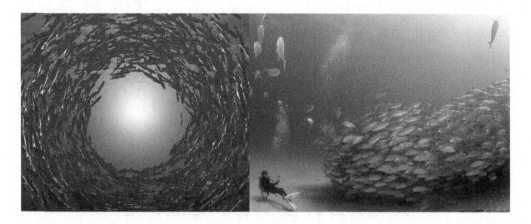

Figure 3.1: Emergent behavior in fish.

A classic example of emergent behavior is an ant colony, which is highly intelligent, even though the individual ants are dumb. Ants have a relatively small repertoire of behaviors that work almost by reflex. For example, they act one way if there is a certain chemical scent in the air, or another way if their neighbor engages in certain body language. But their collective behavior, which emerges from countless interactions between thousands of individual ants, is ingenious. Ant colonies are basically small cities, with highly sophisticated social structures. They build underground nests with many rooms, all of which have specific purposes. Leaf cutter ants have agriculture — they feed from fungus they grow on leaves. Fire ants build living bridges out of their own bodies to cross chasms, and navigate water by arranging themselves into rafts.

Here's a key point about this surprising behavior: **If you only studied the actions of individual ants, you would never guess what they can do as a whole.** What lesson does this hold for studying the body? If you only look at the behavior of muscles, tendons, or joints in isolation, you will miss the big picture of how they work together in real life. Part of the goal of this book is to help build that bigger picture with common sense metaphors that are grounded in complexity science. The big picture on ants is that a whole colony operates as a single unified organism. Each individual ant is like one cell in a large extended body. The big picture on human bodies is that they are like ant colonies. They are made of billions of cells that pursue their own local interests, engaging in simple behaviors like taking in food, repairing damage, repelling invaders, or sending communications to other cells. They have no idea they are part of some larger plan to form an intelligent body. And yet somehow their interactions do exactly that. We are not machines but ecologies, and we operate according to similar logic.

A CROWD OF AGENTS

Complexity science is sometimes called the study of crowd behavior.[8] Investors in a market, birds in a flock, social media users on Facebook, or neurons in a brain are all crowds of agents that make decisions based on the decisions of the other members, which creates a new round of decisions, and so forth. When they interact, the whole can develop a "mind" of its own that might have very different ideas from the minds of the individual members.

All the different cells and organs in the body have their own "intentions," and ways of "thinking" about how to achieve them. Even single cells are smarter than we might imagine.[9] Immune cells discriminate between friend and foe, neurons "decide" whether to communicate with neighbors, and muscle cells respond to load by growing stronger. Nociceptors, the nerve endings that detect potential dangers in the body, may be able to "remember" past instances of trauma.[10] All the different systems in the body have some reason for what they are doing, and we can understand their behavior better if we try to imagine what they want and how they think.[11]

This perspective is missed when we look at body parts as mindless or reflexive. For example, people often stretch their muscles as if they were pieces of meat, ignoring the fact that muscles don't "want" to lengthen past a certain point, and may stiffen to protect themselves from aggressive stretching. A better approach is to "convince" the muscles that a large range of motion is safe. Similarly, if your body wants to rest, it's hard to force it to get moving. Physical activity is easier if we create the conditions that make the body want to get moving, such as finding meaningful activities, favorable social and environmental contexts, or getting more sleep.

NESTING: SUBSYSTEMS AND SUPERSYSTEMS

When crowds of agents interact, they may form subgroups arranged into hierarchies. For example, people gather together in small groups, which may interact to form larger tribes, which may network to form nations. The larger groups emerge from "bottom-up" organization, but they gain some form of "top-down" control over the smaller groups.[12] Most complex adaptive systems are "nested" in this way — they are composed of subsystems, which have their own subsystems, and so forth.[13] Nesting can be seen in governments, large business organizations, and human bodies. A body is a collection of large organ systems, which are composed of individual organs, which are made of cells, which are made of organelles. And bodies are subparts of larger systems like families, communities and economies.

In trying to solve some problem related to movement health — let's say improving functional leg strength — you could turn your attention to any one of these different nested levels. You could look at the micro level, analyzing the size of individual muscles like the quads or hamstrings. You could take a bigger picture perspective, considering the behavior of the nervous system, which controls muscle activation, or the endocrine system, which helps to fuel muscle growth. You could look at the level of the "whole person," where decisions are made about whether to go to the gym, or the societal level, which creates cultural norms about exercise. We can make similar choices about how to analyze problems with pain, obesity, fatigue, or many types of complex diseases.

Each level of analysis may provide unique insights. Advocates of complexity science argue that mainstream medicine has spent too much time at the lower levels, where phenomena are more easily quantified, and not enough at the higher levels, where the interesting events are more qualitative and subjective.[14] As a result, we have neglected the effect of psychology, social systems, and environment on health. A recent editorial in *The Lancet* makes this point: "A radical shift of life sciences funding priorities, away from the biomedical bubble and towards the social, behavioral, and environmental determinants of health, is now needed."[15]

ADAPTIVITY

Complex *adaptive* systems have goals and the means to achieve them. Not all complex systems adapt – clouds don't care which way they get blown by the wind, or even if they disappear into the mist. But living things have a purpose.[16] They want, at a bare minimum, to survive and procreate, and they usually have many other interests as well. They can accomplish these goals only by maintaining a certain set of physiological conditions. These include a full belly, warmth, freedom from infection, and access to refreshing beverages. This state, which is often called homeostasis (and which I call sitting on the couch without the kids around), is always being disturbed by stressors, so the organism needs an appropriate response to restore balance.

These responses often create adaptations that make the system better able to withstand similar stressors in the future. Through continual adaptation, the system evolves over time. Eventually, everything about the system that is in any way interesting is an adaptation to past stressors. The current state of your speed, strength, and agility depends on how you (or your ancestors) moved in the past. **Therefore,** to understand a complex adaptive system, you need to know its history. This is a profound idea, and also common sense. If you want to really comprehend a person or culture, you need to know how they got to be the way they are now. And it is often stated that "nothing in biology makes sense except in light of evolution."[17] With these ideas in mind, this book frequently looks at movement from the perspective of evolution or child development.

NON-LINEARITY

Complex systems are non-linear, meaning their behavior is irregular.[18] For example, the system might have a massive response to a minor stimulus, or little to no response to a major stimulus. Small inputs can produce big outputs, and vice versa.

For example, back pain may be highly disproportionate to mechanical stress. A powerlifter who regularly squats hundreds of pounds with comfort might suddenly keel over when bending to pick up a sock. The healing process might also be nonlinear — pain remains at a constant level for several weeks of rest, and then suddenly fades away. Runners might notice similar patterns with heel or knee pain. Getting better is not a smooth, upward progression, but a jagged line of improvements, coupled with set-backs. If you look at the pattern over days or weeks, you might miss clear signs of an upward trend occurring over months.

Skill acquisition is non-linear. Athletes who practice their sport at a constant rate may experience long plateaus in performance, followed by unexpected quantum leaps.[19] In fact, major improvements are often preceded by brief periods of regression.[20] Parents may notice similar patterns in the development of toddlers. These are all examples of how chaos and order co-exist in a complex system. One feeds off the other. Douglas Hofstadter has an elegant way to describe it: "It turns out that an eerie type of chaos can lurk just behind a facade of order — and yet, deep inside the chaos lurks an even eerier type of order."[21]

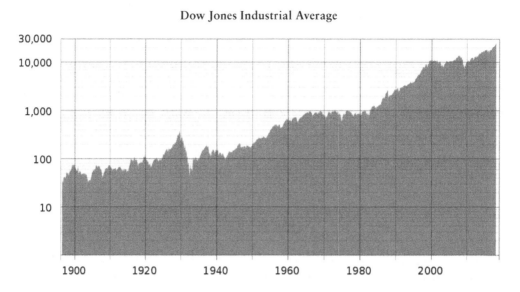

Figure 3.3: Non-linear upward trend of the stock market over a century. Healing patterns may look similar.

Nonlinear behavior is easily observed in many other kinds of complex systems. Traffic jams, tornados, stock market crashes, and political revolutions can occur with little or no warning. These events are often called butterfly effects or black swans, which means they are for all practical purposes unpredictable, even by world-class experts.[22] They are a reminder that we need to remain humble about our ability to fully understand or control the body. No matter how much data we acquire, unexpected events that have a major impact are sure to occur.

FEEDBACK LOOPS

The dynamic behavior of a complex system is driven by connectivity between its different parts. One common pattern of connection is a feedback loop, where the chain of cause and effect leads back to where it started, initiating a new chain of events in slightly modified form. For example, every time we move, this creates sensory feedback, which will prompt a new movement, which will create new sensory feedback, and so forth.

Feedback loops can be negative or positive. Negative feedback promotes stable behavior. It works like this: an input drives the system to move in one direction, and this causes an output that moves the system back to where it came from. For example, here's how you keep your balance in standing: if your center of gravity tilts left, sensory organs detect the movement, and this triggers muscles that pull the body back to the right. Many of the physiological conditions that are required to remain alive — bodyweight, temperature, heart rate, oxygen level — are regulated by negative feedback loops. When some variable gets too high or low, this sends a message that is read by some other part of the body, which responds by acting to restore the state of balance.

Positive feedback loops have the opposite effect — a movement in one direction promotes another move in the *same* direction. This creates extreme change rapidly. Examples are viral videos, cattle stampedes, riots, or stock market crashes. If these vicious cycles don't eventually come under the control of a negative feedback loop, the system will spin out of balance.

In the body, positive feedback loops implement the response to physical emergencies. If we encounter a predator, the body immediately prepares for "fight or flight," which occurs through a cascade of physiological changes.[23] Each one ramps up the energy level of the next, like cheering spectators in a crowd. When we get injured, positive feedback loops quickly increase pain sensitivity: Tissue damage causes inflammation, which increases the sensitivity of nerve endings, which makes them more active, which causes more inflammation, and so forth. This is why several hours after a sprained ankle, the whole area has become massively sensitive. Eventually, negative feedback loops will restore normalcy: Inflammation initiates healing, which reduces damage, which allows more movement, which creates more healing, which reduces inflammation. What if the negative feedback loops don't kick in properly, and the injured area remains stuck in a positive feedback loop? For example, pain prevents movement, which prevents healing, which prevents movement, which reduces fitness, which prevents movement. Playing with movement is a way to escape this loop. Introducing a new stimulus, even a random stimulus, can shake up the system, reactivating negative feedback loops that may have fallen asleep at the switch and need a wake-up call. This dynamic is discussed in more detail in chapter eleven.

VARIABILITY

Complex systems display extreme variability, meaning they are able to assume a near infinite number of different states, even within narrow constraints. Snowflakes all look pretty much the same, but upon close inspection (as the saying goes), no two are alike. Neither are two human footsteps. Even as you walk for miles over even ground at the same pace, you will never step exactly the same way twice. Stride variability is a feature, not a bug of walking. It allows you to transition over different surfaces, shift the stress of movement from one joint to another, and to learn, through trial and error on every step, how to walk more efficiently.

Variability is characteristic of any healthy biological system, and a major source of its functionality, adaptive power, and resilience to stress.[24] In fact, when an organism gets locked into an excessively repetitive pattern, that can be a sign of dysregulation.[25] Thus, reduced or altered variability is associated with poor biological function in a wide variety of contexts, including heart rate[26] and postural balance.[27]

The benefits of variability are easy to understand in the context of economies or ecosystems. Diversity makes the system resilient, by making sure all the eggs aren't in the same basket.[28] In contrast, machines are not variable, and this makes them fragile. When a key part breaks, they stop working. But organic systems continue to function even after serious injury. A car missing one tire can't move at all, but a dog with only three legs gets along pretty well.

[handwritten: HUMANS AREN'T CONSTANT, PREDICTABLE, OR INDEPENDENT]

Variability also benefits coordination, and once again this is quite different from machines. Good engineering of a machine will reduce freedom of movement at the joints to a minimum. If a joint has any "play," that needs to be tightened down. In the body, healthy joints have lots of play, and expert movers actually demonstrate more variability (in some ways) than novices.[29] The benefit of variable movement is having more ways to get the same job done. The quarterback who can throw accurately in many different body postures has an advantage over the guy whose throwing is more robotic. Variability in movement also speeds motor learning, because it allows more experimentation.[30] We'll discuss these issues in greater detail in chapter ten.

ATTRACTORS

The dynamic connections and feedback loops in a complex system push and pull it in different directions. For example, right now there are forces at work in your body — hormones, neural impulses, memories, fears, expectancies — encouraging you to do all sorts of different things: go to the fridge for a snack, lay down and take a nap, go outside for a walk, or log in to Facebook. Which decision gets made? The answer is uncertain, but some outcomes are more statistically likely than others.* An attractor is a state of organization to which a system will tend to gravitate, as a matter of probability.

We can think of attractors as habits, predispositions, or tendencies. Everyone has habits of moving, thinking, and feeling. Some are continually "attracted" into states of fatigue and depression, others to excitement and energetic movement. Habits govern muscular coordination in standing, walking, or running. When infants are born, they haven't yet acquired any functional movement habits. They start out moving semi-randomly, but they are eventually attracted to the classics like reaching, crawling and walking. This is because when they finally stumble upon these highly useful movements, they get positive

---

* The correct answer was (d) go outside for a walk.

feedback. This encourages repetition, which makes the movements even more attractive.[31]

Complexity scientists illustrate attractors with the image of a ball moving over an uneven landscape.[32] Each point in the landscape represents a different possible state for the system, such as feeling good or bad, or running with a heel strike or forefoot strike. The ball is always being pushed and pulled in variable directions by random events, but the position of the ball is not random because the shape of the landscape makes some resting points more likely than others. The ball will be attracted by the wells and repelled from the hills.

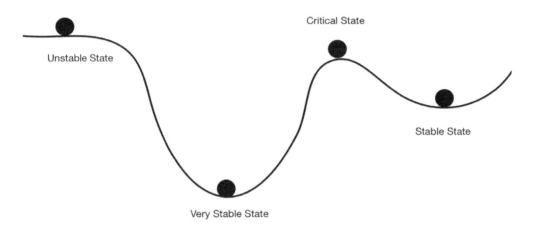

Figure 3.4: An attractor landscape. The system will be attracted to the wells and repelled from hills.

Deep narrow wells represent robust behaviors that will persist over time in many different circumstances. The stability of these behaviors derives from strong negative feedback loops. For example, someone may have a habit of being sedentary because as soon as they start a new exercise program, they get negative feedback, such as fatigue, boredom or pain. We could represent any ingrained habit as a ball sitting in a deep and narrow well. You are literally stuck in a rut.

Flat areas correspond to unstable behavior. This may be due to the system moving into a transitional phase, such as the teenage years for a human, or a new government after a political revolution, or a recent injury. A novice athlete is on a flat area of the movement landscape, and won't find much stability in his performance while exploring new techniques. With practice, certain points on the landscape will deepen into wells, representing the formation of new habits.

Hills on the landscape represent a critical state: the ball is precariously balanced between two opposite outcomes. If the ball moves left, the system returns to normal, but if it moves right, a new normal is established, which is called a phase shift. The system is poised such that everything "hangs in the balance," and small random shifts in fortune can lead to huge differences in final outcome. This is a common-sense idea that can be seen in many different systems — political, economic, social, or biological. In the body, a critical state might be caused by a severe physical or emotional injury. One potential outcome might actually be positive — overcoming a major challenge builds a unique kind of strength and resilience. Or, the trauma could have the opposite effect, leading to a persistent state of sensitivity and fragility. This dynamic can help us understand chronic pain, as we will discuss in greater detail in chapter eleven.

The attractor concept explains numerous phenomena related to fitness. We are all attracted to certain "set points" of muscle, fat, strength and endurance. We can make changes through diet and exercise, but we may gravitate back to a baseline. This will be discussed in greater detail in chapter five. In chapter ten we will discuss how moving with better coordination is about finding and then "deepening" the attractor wells associated with good movement technique. Playing with movement is about escaping well-worn grooves and exploring new territory.

SELF-ORGANIZATION

Complex systems are attracted to states of order, even though there is no central plan. When ants build a nest, there isn't an ant architect looking at a set of blueprints and barking out directions. The nest is built through self-organization, and there is not a single ant that under-stands or even intends the final result. Order emerges spontaneously through widely distributed interactions.

The languages we speak were not designed. They are more like living things that evolved on their own. Efficient markets don't require central planning. We are assured of finding tasty snacks and refreshing beverages in stores not because of government mandate, but through billions of semi-random exchanges between buyers and sellers. Because the source of order is decentralized and bottom-up, it is more robust to unexpected shocks and disturbances.[33]

Self-organization has been described as "order out of chaos," or "order from noise."[34] The system thrives on freedom, and even a bit of randomness, which helps it "explore" different states of organization and find new attractors. Trying to impose strict control over the parts in a self-organizing system can make it less healthy, because it under-mines the basis for adaptation. This can be seen in a wide variety of contexts: excessive governmental regulation of markets; strict parent-ing of children; overly regimented schooling; and the declining coolness of Manhattan.[35] Creativity and dynamism require a certain amount of messiness.

Coordination of the body occurs through self-organization.[36] To move well, you don't need to be told the right way to move, to think about the right way to move, or even have any conscious idea about the right way to move. The role of the conscious mind is mostly lim-ited to directing intention and attention: it makes the decision about what to do (dribble, pass or shoot), and what to focus on (the ball, the opponent, or the basket). But the conscious mind doesn't command the specific muscle contractions used to execute the intention. These emerge from a bottom-up process that is decentralized, embodied in interactions between muscles, joints and sensors all over the body, and the environment. This makes the movement system more robust to disturbance. If the body's organization depended exclusively on top-down direction from the brain, it would completely fall apart as soon as the brain's attention shifted elsewhere. We don't crash the car when we stop thinking about driving. Because coordination lives in inter-actions between many different parts of the body, it continues even when individual members are injured or distracted. Trying to impose strict top-down control over movement (e.g., by consciously bracing the core or firing the glutes) is unlikely to improve organization and may even make it worse. We will discuss this issue in greater detail in chapter ten.

COMPLEX VERSUS COMPLICATED PROBLEMS

You can't control a body in the same way you control a machine. The former problem is properly considered "complex," while the latter is merely "complicated." Although these terms are used interchangeably in everyday life, systems theorists note some profound distinctions.[37]

[Complicated problems have many interrelated parts, but each can potentially be controlled with extreme precision in a top-down man-ner, *provided you have sufficient expertise.*] If you have the know-how, you can send a rocket ship to the moon. And if you don't, you will fail miserably every time you try. With the right medical training, you can perform open heart surgery and save lives. Without it, you will surely kill your patients. For complicated problems, expertise and planning are incredibly important.

Complex problems are different, because expertise isn't necessary or sufficient for success. The classic example is raising a toddler, which is something that complete amateurs succeed at regularly.[38] Toddlers are self-organizing creatures, and will usually do just fine if you give them food, shelter, love and attention. On the other hand, they are also unpredictable, and therefore even an expert in child discipline might fail in getting one to behave. Further, different experts recommend completely different child-rearing strategies, which is very telling. You will not see engineers arguing over what makes planes fly, but there are radically different opinions about the best ways to raise children, stimulate economic growth, or build peaceful relations between nations. When qualified experts have major disagreements over the basics of how to solve a problem, it is most likely complex.

Other examples of complex problems would be eating a nutritious diet, finding motivation to exercise, developing basic movement skills, losing weight, gaining muscle, improving sleep, and minimizing emotional stress. In most cases, expertise will probably help, but will not provide a quantum leap over common sense, individual experimentation, and a strong intention to succeed. Although complicated problems *always* require expert knowledge, solutions to complex problems might be deceivingly simple. You can lose weight by simply eating less and moving more. You can build strength by following any one of many resistance training programs. You can improve endurance by just going out for a comfortable run and building mileage slowly.* Getting these jobs done is not necessarily easy, because you need to find the time and motivation to do them, and you need to deal with dilemmas that arise, such as aches and pains. But the basic plan is not rocket science, and you don't need to complicate it. This is the idea underlying the KISS principle — keep it simple stupid.[39]

We tend to complicate things when we start analyzing, measuring and systematizing. According to Paul Plsek, mechanical thinking believes that "it is necessary to plan and control or there will be chaos."[40] This attitude can be counterproductive, because a controlling mindset may limit the freedom an organic system needs to self-organize. This has been noted by systems theorists in a wide variety of contexts, including public policy, health care, child development, and motor learning. For example, trying to control your posture by sitting up straight will probably make you less comfortable than just allowing your trunk to move naturally. An exercise or rehab program that is full of complicated rules

---

* It is a different story if you want to be a bodybuilder or develop elite level fitness. These problems are complex *and* complicated, and you will need an expert for help.

about technique and sets and reps and times may kill the motivation to comply, which defeats what should be the primary goal.

Because we cannot acquire full knowledge over complex systems, we need to remain humble in our interventions, acting more like a gardener cultivating growth, and less like a craftsman shaping an object.[41] Allison Gopnik uses this metaphor in her book *The Gardener and The Carpenter*, where she argues that a "scientific" approach to parenting tends to discourage the messiness, playfulness and freedom that optimizes childhood development.[42] Similar ideas are found in play-based methods for learning sports skills. The influential systems thinker Donella Meadows has a good line about the indirect methods we need to use in the presence of complexity: "We can't fix complex problems, but we can dance with them."[43]

CONSTRAINTS

Although we can't control a complex system in the same way we program a computer or engineer a machine, we can change the constraints around which it self-organizes. A constraint is defined as a feature of the system or its environment that limits the states the system can assume.[44] Constraints do not so much tell the system what to do, but what it *cannot* do. If your car is in the shop, this constrains your options for getting to work, and you are now more likely to walk. You are free to choose other commuting options, and no one is forcing you to walk, but losing the car gets you more attracted to walking. Here's a more technical explanation of how constraints shape behavior, from Turvey, Kelso and Kugler:

> The order in biological and physiological processes is primarily owing to dynamics . . . **The constraints that arise, both anatomical and functional, serve only to channel and guide dynamics**; it is not that actions are caused by constraints, it is, rather, that some actions are excluded by them.[45]

I think of constraints as like the banks of a river, channeling all the dynamism of the water into a definite shape. The water still has tremendous freedom to move, but within limits. These limits determine the location of ripples, turbulence, or whirlpools. If we rearranged them, the patterns of flow would change. If the banks were removed altogether, the water would have complete freedom, and the river would cease to exist.

Thinking in terms of constraints can be non-intuitive if we assume that behavior always derives from some form of command. For example, if you want your kids to engage in some productive activities, you could command them to go outside or read a book. (Good luck with that.) Or, you could use a strategy based on constraints: take away their computers, TVs and iPads, and tell them they can do whatever they want. The result might be good — they go outside, read a book, or maybe even find a better option you didn't even think of. Self-organizing systems perform best when they are given freedom within appropriate limits, as opposed to being told exactly what to do.

Many personal trainers know this intuitively, using a "constraints-led approach" to teach movement.[46] If a client is squatting with the knees going too far forward, they will ask them to squat in front of a wall, which constrains their movement options, making them attracted to the desired pattern. A soccer coach could command his players to pass more, or he could just change the rules of the practice game, allowing only two touches per possession. Barefoot running is a constraint that encourages people to shorten their stride, increase their cadence, and change their foot strike. In each case, change emerges in a bottom-up fashion. The results are more embodied, authentic, and robust than if they were caused by top-down direction. When changes happen through command, they may be more fragile and impermanent, subject to falling apart as soon as discipline wavers.

Karl Newell's theory of constraints[47] identifies three basic types of constraints related to movement: (1) external constraints, such as features of the environment; (2) individual constraints, such as muscle size and movement habits; and (3) task constraints, such as the need to get the ball over the net in tennis, or touch your butt to a chair in a squat.[48]

The most powerful external constraint is one we generally take for granted: the force of gravity. When an infant is born, it comes into contact with this constraint for the first time. This really limits the infant's options. Every movement needs to resist a downward pull toward the earth. Compared to the womb, there are now far fewer ways to solve the physical problems of life. So every system of the body will start to reorganize. Gravity drives the body toward development of healthy levels of strength, bony integrity, fitness and postural balance. Without it, the baby would remain a poorly formed blob. Indeed, when astronauts go into space, and the constraint of gravity is removed, they start to turn into blobs as well, quickly losing muscle mass and bone density. Many good resistance exercises are basically simulations of an environment with increased gravity. One way or another, human bodies need to be constantly exposed to the constraint of physical challenge to stay organized and healthy.

Internal constraints on movements include the structure of the body and the organization of the nervous system. When these variables change, new opportunities arise, and others are foreclosed. Psychological motivation to accomplish goals is an overlooked internal constraint that has profound effects on movement health. Babies typically want to explore the world and play with toys, and without these goals they would never learn to focus the eyes, control head movement, reach accurately with the hand, and crawl. Over long periods of time, a strong motivation to accomplish a physical goal will transform your body and mind.

Here's why I think all this theoretical stuff is useful: You can think of any effort to improve your movement health as being about playing with the constraints around which your body self-organizes. When a constraint is changed, the dynamics of the system are channeled into a new direction, some predictable, others surprising. How would your movement health change if you modified any one of the following constraints?

- Hip mobility
- Squatting skill
- Tissue quality in the area of an injury
- Back pain
- Motivation to exercise
- Commitment to dance class with your wife
- Social environment
- Job
- Posture
- Body composition
- Residential neighborhood
- Steps per day
- Core strength
- The size of your beer gut
- Fitness routine

The effects of changing some of these variables is relatively obvious — getting out of severe neck pain will lead to major improvements in your movement on multiple levels. Losing 20 pounds of fat will surely make you a faster runner. Other effects will be far less predictable. Will changing your foot strike make you a more efficient runner? Will improving your core strength help with back pain? Does greater flexibility reduce injury risk? Does posture matter? Is back surgery effective? Will stronger legs make you a faster sprinter? Will agility drills make you better at soccer?

In the rest of the book, we will examine the complexities of these and other questions in relation to many different constraints on movement — stress, fitness, structure, posture, mobility, coordination, environment and pain. You can think of these different constraints as dials to turn, variables to tinker with, rules in a game, or different ways to play with movement. We will examine research that might answer which dials are more worth turning, and in what direction. In many cases, although the problems are complex, the solutions are relatively simple.

4

STRESS AND ADAPTATION

That which doesn't kill you makes you stronger.
— FRIEDRICH NIETZSCHE

The dose makes the poison.
—PARACELSUS

Chronic stress contributes to ulcers, insomnia, anxiety, heart disease, depression and chronic pain. Stress can be a killer. But what doesn't kill you can make you stronger, and therefore stress also contributes to health. All exercise, even play, is essentially a form of stress, and can improve strength, endurance, mobility and overall physical function. There is almost nothing about your physical wellness that hasn't been developed by stress, or that couldn't be improved further by more.

"Good stress" produces favorable adaptations, and usually involves some challenge that is short-lived, controllable, and maybe even fun. Examples are roller coaster rides, a quick series of sprints, rock climbing, a long walk, public speaking, or crossword puzzles. Over time, repeated bouts of good stress will make you more healthy, sane and attractive. What doesn't kill you makes you stronger.

"Bad stress" is usually prolonged, unpleasant, excessive, and largely beyond your control. Examples are traffic jams, insomnia, abusive relationships, car crashes, and bad musicals. Over time, or even in an instant if the stress is extreme (e.g., a really bad musical), these events can overwhelm the system, or slowly deplete vital resources, leaving you weaker and less adaptable. This helps explain why exercise is generally healthy, while chronic emotional stress is not.

But this general rule can only take us so far. A particular form of stress might be good for one person and bad for another. The same exercise program can build up one athlete and break down another. And the same crappy job and diet will have vastly different effects on different people. There is no one-size-fits-all recipe for exercise, sleep, or diet. Finding the best solution requires exploration of a vast landscape of possibilities. Despite this inherent variability, some common patterns emerge. To see them clearly, it helps to zoom out in our perspective, so we can see some links between mental and physical that are otherwise invisible.

STRESS AND PHYSICAL CHALLENGE

Stress is the body's physiological response to a challenge.[1] A stressor is something that knocks you out of a desired state of balance, and the stress response is the body's attempt to restore it. Imagine encountering a lion while strolling through the African savanna. The lion is a stressor, and when you perceive it you will immediately experience stress— a cascade of physiological changes intended to help you survive what appears to be a life-threatening emergency. You are now prepared for "fight or flight."

What physiological changes occur and why? You will feel terrified, which motivates you to make self-protection your top priority, as opposed to say, continuing to chat with your friend. You may experience tunnel vision, to get you focused on what's important. Your heart rate, breathing, and muscle tension will elevate to prepare for intense physical work. This work requires fuel, so your blood sugar levels are increased, as is blood pressure, to speed delivery of fuel to muscles. Your perception of pain is drastically reduced, so you can continue to move even if you are seriously injured.

You might also get a dry mouth. How does this help fight a lion? This is a side effect of another important aspect of the stress response — the shifting of resources away from bodily functions that are not directly related to immediate survival. Digestion of food requires a lot of energy, so all related activities, including the production of saliva, are temporarily put on hold. So are various other projects related to physical growth, sexual reproduction, repair of tissue damage, or fighting infections. These forward-looking functions are important, but there is no harm in delaying them for a few minutes until you reach safety. It doesn't make sense to worry about minor house repairs in the middle of an earthquake.

When the emergency is over, the body will shift out of "fight or flight" and into "rest and digest." This is the pleasurable state of feeling drowsy after a tasty Thanksgiving dinner with friends and family, or walking on the beach at sunset on vacation. We enter this state when there are no immediate threats, no reason for vigilance, and all signs point to the presence of shelter, social support, food, and refreshing beverages.[2] Physiological resources are now diverted from crisis management to long-term building projects. "Liquid" energy in the form of blood sugar is reinvested into cellular storage banks. The immune system becomes more active to fight infections and heal tissue damage. Hormonal balance reorganizes to promote muscle growth and sexual drive. All these changes represent an "optimistic" perspective. The body perceives it will survive for more than the next half hour, so it starts planning for the future, by building more muscle, healing injuries, and maybe even raising some kids.[3] And then, when another lion shows up, these projects are temporarily put on hold, until the emergency passes, and more future investment can be done.

This "surviving" versus "thriving" dichotomy illustrates the extreme ends of the stress spectrum. Most of life is spent somewhere in between, where nuanced trade-offs are always being made, minute by minute, even second by second. Stress is not just for emergencies — you need just a touch to walk up the stairs or get out of bed in the morning. The sympathetic branch of the autonomic nervous system gets more active when you need to meet a challenge, while the parasympathetic promotes relaxation. At each moment in time, the system is adjusting sympathetic or parasympathetic "tone" so that the body is optimally tuned for the circumstance.[4] Every time you exhale, you relax just a little bit compared to the inhale, which is more invigorating.

Thus, a healthy stress response system is constantly adjusting its level of activation or relaxation. Balance is maintained by constant communication between the nervous system, immune system, and endocrine system. This is achieved through chemical mediators such as hormones, cytokines, and neurotransmitters.[5] The hub of this communication is the brain, especially the "HPA axis," a web of connections between the hypothalamus, pituitary gland and adrenal glands.[6] This system is working hard when we are under a lot of stress, and chronic over-activation can lead to wear and tear on the involved organs, depletion of the chemical mediators necessary for communication, and resulting imbalance in the system as a whole.[7] When balance is disturbed, the body may become attracted to a more protective state, making it harder to sleep, relax or enjoy life. This is unpleasant for a few hours, and when it persists for months or years, it can contribute to serious health problems, such as depression, anxiety, obesity, chronic fatigue and pain.[8] One of the main sources of chronic stress is emotional, which as we will see, causes a physiological reaction that is very similar to how we respond to physical threats.

EMOTIONAL STRESS

The basic physiology governing the human stress response evolved tens of millions of years ago and is shared by all vertebrate animals.[9] Its original purpose was to deal with physical challenges. But in social

animals, and especially humans, emotional challenges also activate
the stress response, even if they do not involve an immediate physical
threat.[10] Thus, sitting in a tense job interview creates a similar physiological response to walking through a dangerous neighborhood at
night. This is unfortunate. It makes perfect sense for our bodies to prepare for physical emergencies by increasing blood pressure, breathing
faster, flooding the bloodstream with blood sugar, increasing muscular
tension and shutting down immune function and digestion. But when
we are sitting in a traffic jam trying to get to our child's baseball game,
these conditions are not very helpful at all. In his excellent book, *Why
Zebras Don't Get Ulcers*, Stanford biologist Robert Sapolsky describes
why many stress responses in the modern world are "maladaptive."

> If your blood pressure rises to 180/100 when you're sprinting
> away from a lion, you are being adaptive, but if it is 180/100
> every time you see the mess in your teenager's bedroom, you
> could be heading for cardiovascular disaster.[11]

In the modern world, we have opportunities to feel emotional stress all
day, from jobs, mortgages, dinner parties, and distant events over which
we have no control, such as presidential elections and global warming.
These ever-present emotional challenges may create an "evolutionary
mismatch" for our ancient stress systems.[12] They evolved to deal with
challenges that are physical and intermittent, not emotional and constant.
This is why the former is generally good for us, and the latter not so
good at all. Chronic emotional stress probably plays a role in heart disease, obesity, hypertension, diabetes and other "diseases of civilization."[13]
Stress is also known to be a risk factor for depression, anxiety, gastroin-
testinal problems, Alzheimer's, and other chronic health conditions.[14]

Why does chronic stress cause so many different health problems?
Part of the answer is that a good stress response is fundamental to life,
and therefore involves almost every major system in the body — cardiovascular, immune, nervous, endocrine, etc. Chronic stress therefore has
the potential to overload the body in multiple ways.

STRESS AND ADAPTATION

Now that we've talked about the costs of getting too much of the wrong kind of stress, let's appreciate the amazing benefits of getting the right amount of the right kind. Everything about your body that is well-organized got that way because of prior experiences with stress. The strength of every bone, muscle and tendon derives from adaptations that were initiated by challenges in handling a physical load. Every skill you possess — the ability to stand up straight, walk around, or play a sport — was learned during past failures in finding solutions to movement problems. Your immune system can fight infections because you frequently got sick. All of your cognitive and emotional resilience is built on lessons learned from facing mental obstacles. Thus, every aspect of your movement health depends on your past history of facing stress. So let's look at some basic principles of stress adaptation, so we can put these facts to good use.

Hans Selye is a physiologist who articulated some general principles explaining how living things adapt and grow. His "general adaptation syndrome" described three basic phases. In the alarm phase, the organism detects a threat that disturbs a desired state of balance. In the resistance phase, resources are mobilized to meet the threat and/or adapt to similar future challenges. The exhaust phase describes what happens if stress continues to mount, overwhelming the organism's capacity to respond, causing disease and eventually death. According to the logic of his model, Selye distinguished two kinds of stress. Eustress (good stress) creates adaptations that make you strong and healthy, and distress (bad stress) overwhelms you, making you sick and weak.

Selye's ideas have been significantly modified since they were developed, but the basic framework remains highly influential, and useful in explaining how athletes train to become fitter, and even how they learn movement skills.[15] It also fits with basic concepts about the adaptivity of complex systems. Here are some general principles relevant to the development of movement health.

Overload

A stressor will cause an adaptation only if it exceeds a certain threshold of intensity and frequency. In the world of physical training, this is called the overload principle.[16] For example, if you carry a few grocery bags from the car to the refrigerator, this technically "stresses" the muscles, but not enough for them to become bigger or stronger. Frequency matters as well. Carrying many grocery bags at the same time (one of my favorite challenges) can be an intense stimulus, but it would need to be repeated many times before it caused a meaningful change in strength. Fitness or movement skill cannot be built in a day (although it is quite easy to get injured in just a day).

To understand why, remember that your body has been adapting to movement stress your whole life. Therefore, your current level of fitness and coordination is a reflection of what your body "thinks" is an optimal solution to life's physical challenges. Your muscles are the size they are, and not larger, because it would be costly to build and maintain a bigger set, and the body doesn't want to pay these costs unless it's necessary.[17] To encourage a change, you need to send a strong message that the current state of the body is not getting the job done. The same considerations apply to building denser bones, thicker tendons, more lung capacity, and even better movement skills.

Therefore, the degree of stress that will drive an adaptation must be great enough to create a minor crisis. The squeaky wheel gets the grease. At the same time, the crisis must not be so extreme that it causes injury. **Therefore, the level of stress that will promote beneficial adaptation should be in the "goldilocks zone" — not too much and not too little.** This important rule will be restated throughout the book.

Recovery

Stress doesn't cause adaptation until the stress is over and recovery begins. Recall that during stress, the body is hormonally optimized to deal with emergencies, not start new building projects. Thus, you can't adapt if you don't recover. Nor can you learn. The process of learning new skills starts during focused practice, but is consolidated in downtime like sleep and daydreaming. Thus, the basic formula for improving movement health is this:

$$\text{Challenge} + \text{Rest} = \text{Growth}$$

Diminishing returns

Complex systems can only adapt within certain limits, and when they approach them, change is harder. Therefore, training has diminishing returns. The better you get, the harder you have to work to get better still.

When you start a new activity, your performance will improve quickly, even with a lax training regimen. Novice strength trainers will progress their lifts every week, provided they show up at the gym and put in a little effort. If you take up tennis, you don't *need* lessons to get better, you just need to play. And beginning runners will quickly improve their endurance by following any one of many different programs. At the novice stage, just showing up is 80% of the battle, and if you do that, the adaptations will come easily. These quick improvements are sometimes called "newbie gains." They are like the low-hanging fruit of movement health. One of the practical messages of this book is that you should pick as much low-hanging movement health fruit as possible. Another is that play is often sufficient to pick that fruit with a minimum of effort.

As you progress to the intermediate stage of fitness or skill, improvements come slower, and at a higher price. To avoid plateaus, you need to increase the volume and intensity of your training. The quality of your program will probably require some improvement as well. Tennis players may need lessons; weightlifters and runners might need to quantify their training, so they can be sure it is progressing. Another feature of the intermediate stage is that the window between too little and too much exercise stress is growing smaller. The "goldilocks" zone is now harder to find. It is therefore common for intermediate athletes to develop overuse injuries. (Especially if they are in middle age!)

If you reach an elite level of performance, you can't make additional progress without subjecting yourself to a tremendous volume and intensity of physical and emotional stress. The goldilocks zone is now extremely narrow. You are continually on the verge of getting injured, systematically fatigued, or emotionally burnt out. Adequate rest and recovery are now of utmost importance, and you probably can't get enough if you have a day job. On the other hand, if you rest too much and back off on your training, you won't get sufficient stress to maintain your adaptations, and your skills and fitness will regress. This is because your body in some sense does not "want" to be in a state that allows world-class performance. This implies an allocation of resources that is highly specialized — too many eggs in one basket. Not surprisingly, elite performance requires a lot of work, and just playing around won't get the job done. However, **because of the importance of minimizing unnecessary emotional stress, the workload should include as many elements of play as reasonably possible.**

Specificity

We adapt to the *specific* challenges we encounter, not challenges in general. If your leg muscles are stressed by squats, they will get stronger, but your arms will not. If you practice catching a ball, you will develop ball-catching skills, but you won't get better at surfing or guitar. Although adaptations are specific, they may still provide general benefit. Bigger leg muscles might improve your performance in many different activities, such as running, jumping or kicking. Learning to catch a baseball will probably teach you something about how to catch a football, or hit a tennis ball, provided you haven't done these things very much before. But many other adaptations have far less "carry-over" to other activities than you might imagine. Learning to balance on an unstable surface while lifting weight is not likely to improve your overall coordination, or even your balance on a stable surface. A consistent program of cycling will have limited transfer to running, even though they both train aerobic endurance. The amount of carryover that any form of training has for a particular sport is a highly complex topic, one that is the subject of frequent debate by sport scientists. Even seemingly simple questions, like whether bigger leg muscles will make you a better sprinter, are less certain than you might imagine. This book will not address those debates, which are highly specific and contextual, but it will offer some (admittedly speculative) opinions about the kinds of fitness and skills that support what is sometimes called "GPP" — general physical preparedness.

Reversibility

Fitness adaptations have a "use it or lose it" nature. When the stress that creates them is removed, the adaptations slowly fade. That being said, muscles seem to retain some "memory" of their prior level of strength and endurance, making it easier for them to recover their past abilities after they are lost.[18] Memories related to motor skills are far more permanent. Even after decades of neglect, we don't forget how to ride a bike.

Individuality

Teenage boys with no training history will gain muscle quickly even on a crummy program. A middle-aged man will not adapt as easily (trust me). This may be due to different hormonal profiles, which as we said earlier are highly involved in the stress response. But there are many other reasons that people adapt to stress differently, and this should be considered the rule rather than the exception. In fact, some people seem to be "non-responders" to certain exercise programs. For example, a study might find that a group of people on average got fitter after biking a few times a week, but that some people in the group didn't improve fitness at all. However, other studies have shown that people who don't respond to one exercise program will do fine with another. For example, in a study comparing endurance versus sprint training on a bike, everyone adapted to one of the programs, even though many did not respond to both.[19]

SLEEP AND STRESS

Sleep and stress have an antagonistic relationship. Sleep helps fight the negative effects of excess stress, and excess stress makes it hard to sleep. Further, lack of sleep tends to create its own set of challenges that create further stress. Many readers will recognize this horrible vicious cycle from experience.

A good night's sleep can be incredibly restorative. During sleep, muscles rebuild, tissues are repaired, infections are fought, and memories and skills are consolidated. Neurotoxins are literally washed from the brain.[20] Sleep deprivation denies these benefits and is therefore one of the most potent stressors that can be applied to the human body. It is literally a form of torture. It is therefore not surprising that poor sleep correlates with all sorts of negative health outcomes, including impaired immune function, cardiovascular disease, high blood pressure, diabetes, obesity, reduced cognitive function, depression and anxiety, and all-cause mortality.[21]

There is a strong association between insomnia and chronic pain. This relationship is partly explained by the fact that pain makes it harder to sleep. But it's also true that reduced sleep can exacerbate pain. In fact, poor sleep is a better predictor of pain than vice versa. The mechanism is probably that insomnia impairs physiological processes (such as pain inhibition, discussed more in Chapter 11), that are important in the prevention of chronic pain.[22] Several studies have found that insomnia causes symptoms similar to fibromyalgia, including increased pain sensitivity.[23] Further, people who are in "sleep debt" can reduce their pain sensitivity by extending their sleep.[24]

Sleep is also connected to physical performance. Although the research is mixed, it appears that chronic sleep deprivation has negative effects on endurance, cognitive performance, and mood stability.[25] You can predict injury in high school athletes by looking at how many hours they sleep. One study found that athletes who slept less than eight hours per night were 1.7 times more likely to get injured than athletes who slept more than eight hours.[26] In another study, basketball players who increased their sleep to ten hours per night improved sprinting, shooting accuracy, and mental well-being.[27]

STRESS AND PERCEPTION

One of the complexities of stress is that it depends on perception. To illustrate, let's return to the lion example. What if you thought for some reason that the lion was not dangerous? (This is not implausible – YouTube is full of people approaching dangerous animals as if they were friendly dogs.) Maybe you have good reason to be calm — you have knowledge of lion behavior and can see that this one is not in the mood for eating people. Or you are carrying a high-powered rifle and know how to use it. In either case, your heart rate might barely elevate. On the other hand, imagine you had a past traumatic experience with a lion attack. Seeing a lion, even from the safety of a tour bus, might cause a panic attack.

The lesson is that stress depends on subjective perception, which in turn depends on past experience, expectation, and knowledge about your skills and abilities. If you don't perceive a challenge, there is no stress response. And if you do perceive a challenge, even if one does not exist, your body will react. Personally, my hands will literally sweat when I watch videos of daredevils playing on the tops of skyscrapers. The "mind/body connection" is often considered mystical or profound. But it should be quite obvious that fear is subjective, and that stress is in the eye of the beholder.

The brain determines what is threatening, and is therefore "the key organ" in the stress response.[28] The emotional regions of the brain are the first to detect a threat, so stress is heavily affected by mood.[29] For example, negative emotion can increase pain, inflammation levels, and healing time after an injury.[30]

Prior life experience may have a dramatic effect on threat perception. In post-traumatic stress disorder, the stress response systems become dysregulated, leading to persistent hyper-vigilance and sensitivity to innocuous stimuli. Trauma that occurs during childhood seems to have a particularly strong effect and increases risk for a wide variety of psychological and physical health problems. Conversely, a positive childhood tends to dampen the stress response, and encourages healthy risk-taking. For example, rats who receive strong maternal care seem to be "neophilic" — more willing to explore novel environments.[31]

Chronic stress is linked to structural and functional changes in various brain areas, including volume reduction in the prefrontal cortex and limbic system. Similar changes are seen in the brains of people who are depressed or suffer from severe emotional trauma.[32] In PTSD, atrophy of the hippocampus has been reported, which is probably caused by chronic imbalance in the HPA axis.[33]

STRESS AND SPORT

The role of subjective perception in the stress response has major implications for how we train to promote movement health or sport performance. It means that we must consider psychological factors, not just objective variables like sets and reps. According to sports scientist John Kiely, who applies a complex systems perspective in training athletes, subjectivity is a commonly neglected training variable:

> ... the magnitude of the stress response is not directly dependent on the magnitude of the stressor. Instead **it is the emotional resonance attached to the stressor** —the registering of

the stimulus as threatening or benign; as stimulating or anxiety-inducing— that ultimately dictates the extent of the stress defences mobilized . . . Accordingly, **the response to any given stressor is heavily modulated by subjective perception.**[34]

High levels of stress have been shown to impair athletic performance, recovery, fitness gains from exercise, and wound healing.[35] Triathletes are known for their ability to inhibit pain perception, but this superpower is reduced under stressful conditions.[36] There is evidence that chronic emotional stress predicts injury.[37] For example, athletes with preseason anxiety are more likely to get hurt.[38] Stress after an injury predicts greater difficulty in return to play. These findings are especially notable in light of the inability of various biomechanical screening tests to accurately predict injury risk. (See Chapter 10 for more.) Interestingly, subjective measures of stress level, which are obtained by simply asking an athlete about their readiness to train, are better reflections of actual training load than objective measures like hormone levels or markers of inflammation.[39]

These facts also have implications for planning a detailed training program. If you are running a marathon in six months, does it make sense to decide today exactly what a training session should look like three months from now? We know it should probably be harder than the one you did today, but can you be sure it should be precisely 10 miles at 8 min/mile pace?

Periodization is a sophisticated method of athletic training where the overall load is sequenced in a very precise manner. A series of training "blocks" or "cycles" are determined weeks or months in advance, each intended to cause specific fitness adaptations. For example, one block may prioritize aerobic endurance, and another will focus on strength or power. The plan might provide high levels of detail on the exact quantities of work to be done on each day. Trainers like John Kiely are skeptical about the ability of these programs to forecast ahead of time exactly what kinds of physical stress will best promote an athlete's fitness on

Should have pt.s "check in" regarding readiness to train to modulate exercises for the day

a given day.[40] There are simply too many random variables involved, such as sleep, injury, recovery, and motivation. When these are considered, the plan must change. Therefore, good training programs must tinker and play around with training variables, and account for subjective factors like perceived readiness to train.

Although research shows that periodization may be helpful, there is little evidence that one form of periodization works better than another. The one thing every good plan has in common is gradually progressing the level of stress, while making sure the kind of stress is varied. Thus, it may be that the exact order and specifics of the training variations are less important than the fact that they exist.[41] Like all complex adaptive systems, humans benefit from exposure to variable stresses, which gives them a more comprehensive set of adaptations. Changes in training prevent boredom and staleness and inject some randomness into a system that needs a bit of chaos to drive creativity. A plan is useful, but it must be a flexible plan, one that acknowledges the complexity of stress. These basic rules apply not only to athletes, but to people looking to adapt to the stresses of everyday life.

PLAYING WITH STRESS

Stress is multidimensional and complex, so how do we find simple ways to think about it? The stress vulnerability model uses the metaphor of a bucket to visualize how different kinds of stress add up on a daily basis.[42] Similar concepts are sometimes used to manage an athletic training load, or help people treat chronic pain.[43]

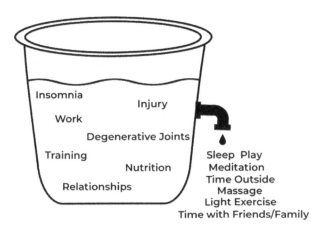

Figure 4.1: A bucket of stressors.

The bucket is filled with stressors, both emotional and physical. These might relate to exercise, work, travel, relationships, finances, sleep, or illness. As long as your bucket is not overflowing, you can adequately respond to each stressor, and fully recover before new ones arise. In fact, you may grow stronger as a result of challenging yourself at the right level, especially when there is adequate chance to recover, and the stresses are of the kind that we evolved to adapt to, such as physical activity. The right amounts and sources of stress can increase the size of the bucket, representing a higher level of general health, resilience and work capacity.[44]

But if the bucket overflows, you will immediately get some negative feedback — perhaps pain, fatigue, or anxiety that does not quickly subside after a reasonable recovery time. If your bucket continues to overflow, your resilience will start to suffer. The size of the bucket will effectively become smaller, meaning that you have less adaptive capacity. Over longer periods of time, chronic stress may awaken dormant vulnerabilities, both genetic or environmental, to chronic pain, fatigue, anxiety, autoimmune disease, or insomnia.[45] In the context of exercise, excessive physical stress may cause "overtraining," which can impair performance, decrease motivation, and elevate the risk of injury and psychological burnout. A workout routine that you formerly handled with ease might seem impossible to complete, or will produce an over-use injury. Back pain that you thought was "fixed" may reemerge.

The bucket analogy is useful in illustrating the multi-causal nature of stress-related symptoms. When back pain suddenly shows up, we are tempted to blame it on the last minor stressor that affected it, such as a soft bed in a hotel. This is like blaming your bankruptcy on the last latte you bought before your account finally went into the red. Thinking in terms of the bucket provides a more expansive view of cause and effect.

OR SINKING BOAT

Each person has their own bucket size, a unique set of stressors to fill it, and a particular sensitivity to each stressor. Some of these differences are due to genetics, others to past history, others to random environmental and social circumstances. As mentioned earlier, past experiences with trauma, especially at a young age, seem to have a particularly strong effect on stress sensitivity, and can explain why some people are easily overwhelmed. Others have a genetic predisposition to certain kinds of illnesses, and they are like kindling for a fire that may or may not be lit by excess stress.

To prevent the bucket from continually overflowing, you need to either reduce the volume of one or more stressors, or somehow increase the quality of your recovery time. Not all free time is equally restorative. Spending time with family and friends, getting outdoors into natural settings, or engaging in meditative activities are all good options for draining the bucket. There are certain physical activities that might check all these boxes, especially those that people tend to self-select while on a relaxing vacation: hiking, biking, swimming, or yoga. In fact, playful physical activity is probably one of the best ways to expose yourself to physical challenge in a healthy way, so you can become stronger, more resilient, and better able to handle other forms of stress.

Of course, the type and intensity of physical challenge that will most effectively fill your bucket without overflowing will require some experimentation to find. When I was in my 30s and working as an attorney, I found that a hard game of squash after work actually served to release some of the tension I built up during the day. Now at age 50, a squash match is still fun but not exactly restorative — a far better choice would be a long walk.

Playing with movement in the context of stress means tinkering with these kinds of considerations — identifying bad stresses you might never have noticed (especially emotional), and finding good stresses that build you up without breaking down. The goal is to slowly grow the size of your bucket over time, so that you increase your resilience and general function.

5

FITNESS

Walking is man's best medicine.
—HIPPOCRATES

*Me thinks that the minute my legs begin to
move my thoughts begin to flow.*
—HENRY DAVID THOREAU

In the early seventies, Jonah Barrington won six British Opens in squash, mostly on the strength of his supreme endurance. At the time, there wasn't much popular interest in fitness, and it wasn't unusual for professional athletes to spend more time off the field smoking and drinking than lifting weights in the gym. But Barrington believed in the benefits of brutal workouts. He took pride in a sado-masochistic level of discipline, and declared himself to be the "fittest man in the world."

In the late '70s and '80s, fitness became trendy, and activities like jogging, aerobics and bodybuilding gained broad popularity. By the 1990s, people started to get interested in "extreme" sports. In 1997, *Outside* magazine named Mark Allen, a six-time Iron Man winner, the "fittest man on earth." In 2000, CrossFit got started, and its killer workouts quickly developed a cult-like following. CrossFit gyms grew in numbers from only one to more than 13,000 in just a decade. In 2007, the CrossFit Games established a formal competition in the "sport of fitness." Rich Froning was the winner from 2011-2014, and during that time was frequently hailed as the "fittest man on earth."

So who was actually the fittest? The best answer is . . . that the question isn't very good. Asking who is "fittest" is roughly analogous to asking who is the most physically "prepared." It begs the question: prepared for what? Cold exposure? A punch to the gut? A zombie apocalypse? Since there are many different kinds of physical stress, there are also many different kinds of fitness. Froning was perfectly fit for CrossFit competitions, as was Allen for triathlons, and Barrington for squash. None of them was even close to being optimally prepared for elite competition in the other disciplines.

This is why fitness is divided into sub categories. The simplest distinction is strength versus endurance. There are many other commonly used categories, including power, strength-speed, speed-strength, aerobic, anaerobic, mobility, etc. Because fitness is to some extent specific, there can be tradeoffs in developing it. The huge muscles that allow Froning to repeatedly power clean 200-pound barbells will make him easily fatigued on the squash court. Barrington's hip flexibility is an asset in squash, which requires lots of deep lunging, but would probably work against his efficiency as a runner, where stiff hamstrings provide better economy of motion. Therefore, becoming more fit in one area has the potential to make you less fit in another.

But these tradeoffs usually occur only when you are approaching an advanced level of performance, which requires you to be a specialist. For most people, increased fitness in one area will benefit performance in others. Stronger legs can make you a more efficient runner. Better hip mobility can add numbers to your squat. And good aerobic capacity is a solid foundation for almost anything you do physically. Thus, although Froning, Allen, and Barrington were specialists, each man had excellent general fitness, and would be expected to perform quite well in a wide range of activities. You would definitely pick any of them to be on your flag football team, or to move your furniture, or to help you survive a zombie apocalypse.

Were these men also excellent models of movement health? They were certainly incredibly healthy people, otherwise they could not have withstood the extreme and varied demands of their sports. Each had a very large "bucket" into which they poured tremendous amounts of stress. But were they healthy because of their training or in spite of it? Extreme training loads create extreme levels of stress, and this may come with a price that can include chronic pain, fatigue, depression, or poor immune function.[1] Fitness is an essential dimension of movement health, but extreme fitness implies an imbalanced allocation of physiological resources. This chapter is about the complex relationship between physical activity, fitness, health, and performance. You can think of it as a rough map for a vast landscape.

PHYSICAL ACTIVITY IS INCREDIBLY GOOD FOR YOU

Fitness has not always been so popular that people argued online about who is the fittest person on Earth. In the middle of the twentieth century, Western medicine had little appreciation for the connection between a sedentary lifestyle and disease. But in 1949, the Scottish epidemiologist Jerry Morris made an interesting discovery comparing the health of different employees on double decker buses in London. Morris found it interesting that the drivers, who sat all day, had higher rates of cardiovascular disease than the conductors, who did their jobs standing, and also repeatedly climbed the stairs. Further study by Morris found that postal workers who delivered mail by foot had fewer heart attacks than clerks sitting behind desks.

Morris' work helped to initiate rapid growth in research examining the health benefits of physical activity. The results have been striking.

Physical activity is now considered one of the "big four" lifestyle factors (along with smoking, nutrition and drug abuse) that have major effects on health. In 2015, the Academy of Medical Royal Colleges put out a report summarizing the benefits of exercise, calling it both a "miracle cure" and a "wonder drug."[2] The report observes that regular exercise can prevent dementia, type 2 diabetes, some cancers, depression, heart disease and other common serious conditions — reducing the risk of each by at least 30%. This is better than many drugs. The report summarizes evidence that physical activity can prevent or treat symptoms from at least twenty chronic conditions, including:

- Hyperlipidemia
- High blood pressure
- Metabolic syndrome
- Diabetes
- Obesity
- Anxiety
- Depression
- Dementia/cognitive decline
- Schizophrenia
- Insomnia
- Digestion
- Parkinson's
- Multiple sclerosis
- Osteoarthritis
- Rheumatoid arthritis
- Chronic pain
- Cancer
- COPD

Similar studies have concluded that a sedentary lifestyle is a primary cause of 36 diseases, and that exercise is an effective treatment to prevent them.[3] Numerous experts have observed that if exercise came in a pill, it would be the most effective and widely prescribed medicine ever developed. Here are a few specific examples of relevant findings.

Low back pain

General exercise, meaning whatever exercise you enjoy, is an effective treatment for low back pain. Most studies find that it works just as well as specific medical interventions, such as chiropractic adjustment, massage, motor control exercise prescribed by a physical therapist, core strengthening, or many forms of surgery.[4]

Osteoarthritis of the knee

Contrary to popular belief, running does not accelerate knee osteo-arthritis through "wear and tear." In fact, it improves function and reduces pain.[5] Resistance training improves pain in osteoarthritis of the knee (and hip) as much as NSAIDS. Aerobic training works just as well as a steroid injection.[6]

Cognitive ability and dementia

Physical activity reduces the risk for dementia, and improves symptoms of dementia, even one year after the exercise program ends.[7] Aerobic exercise has been shown to improve memory, and to increase hippo-campal volume.[8] In one study, elderly adults increased gray and white matter volume after six months of aerobic exercise through walking.[9]

Illness from cold and flu

Several randomized controlled trials have shown that moderate aerobic exercise (daily brisk walking) can cut sick days in half.[10]

Depression and anxiety

The effects of exercise on symptoms of depression are moderate, but probably as good as talk therapy or drug treatment. Several studies have found that exercise improves symptoms of anxiety, but it is not known if the effects are long term.[11]

Overall mortality

A recent analysis of data from more than 60,000 respondents found that people exercising 1-2 times per week had a 30% reduction in all-cause mortality compared to those who got no exercise. There was a 35% reduction for people who exercised 3-5 times.[12]

PHYSICAL ACTIVITY AS
A KEY CONSTRAINT ON HEALTH

How does physical activity work to improve so many different systems in the body? It is not surprising that exercise would strengthen a muscle, but a link to improved cognition is less intuitive. Part of the explanation is that humans, and indeed all animals, are fundamentally in the business of producing movements. All the physiological activity going on under the hood — digestion, metabolism, respiration, circulation, even cognition and emotion — is ultimately in service of producing externally directed movements that help with survival and procreation. From a Darwinian perspective, nothing else really matters. Movement is always the end goal, and is therefore directly connected to every system of importance in the body. When those systems are challenged to help you move, they will adapt to get better at it. If they are not used in this capacity, they may fall into disrepair.

Physical activity is therefore a key constraint that organizes the body, keeping it attracted to states of order that are healthy and functional. Without this constraint in place, the system tends towards entropy and chaos. Everything goes haywire without movement to provide order. To see this most clearly, we can look at circumstances where the body doesn't do *any* muscle work for extended periods of time. Despite the sedentary nature of modern life, there are relatively few circumstances where muscle activity is completely eliminated. When it is, the negative effects are quick and dramatic. Let's consider a few extreme examples — astronauts, bed rest, and joint immobilization.

Astronauts have the opportunity to be extremely lazy, because the weightless environment eliminates the need for even minor muscle work. On Earth, the simple act of standing upright requires constant effort by the postural muscles. But in space, these muscles take a relaxing vacation. As a result, they very quickly start to shrivel like grapes. Astronauts can lose up to 20% of their muscle mass in as little as 10 days. The effects on bone density are equally dramatic. Astronauts lose

1.5% of their bone mass every month, which is about 60 times the rate associated with normal aging. After four months in space, they lose so much bone density they will not regain it for two years.[13]

Why the extreme reaction to a little vacation from physical activity? It seems the body needs constant reminders that muscles and bones serve important functional purposes and should not be cannibalized for energy. When the constraint of gravity is gone, the system immediately becomes disorganized, like a river without any banks. The muscular system does not "know" what to do when normal levels of physical challenge aren't there.

Bed rest is another example of what happens to the body when it stops moving. After about a month of lying in bed, inactive muscles lose about half their strength, ligaments lose 60% of their ability to bear load, and tendons lose significant stiffness. If joints are immobilized in a short position for two to three weeks, adhesions may start to form that impede full range of motion. By six months, surgery may be required to break them.[14]

MOVEMENT AS A NUTRIENT

Although movement is sometimes called medicine, I think a better metaphor is one recommended by Katy Bowman and Nick Tuminello: movement is like food. Nutrients in food are beneficial when consumed in some goldilocks amount — not too much and not too little. For example, you need a minimum dose of iron to avoid anemia, but too much is toxic. Many kinds of inputs to the body follow this pattern, even water. The dose makes the poison, and the cure as well. With physical activity, some minimum amount is essential, too much is toxic, and in between there is a broad range of happy mediums.

Another analogy between food and movement is that you need a well-balanced diet of many different nutrients, all of which have a different optimum dose. If you have a deficiency in Vitamin A, it won't help to double up on the Vitamin B. The same is true of physical activity. The bench press is a fine exercise, but if that's all you ever did, you would become deficient in other areas of physical function.

A BALANCED MOVEMENT DIET

If movement is a nutrient, how much do you need to be healthy? And what kinds? Part of the answer is, of course … it depends. A deconditioned 65-year-old with knee pain should not have the same exercise plan as a fit 20-year-old athlete. In fact, two deconditioned 65-year-olds with knee pain might benefit from completely different programs. Thus, optimal fitness programs can only be found by exploring a wide landscape of potential options. That being said, some parts of the landscape are more worth exploring than others. To get a rough idea where they are, we can look to two sources of data: (1) formal recommendations from government health groups; and (2) research analyzing the physical activity of hunter-gatherers living in natural environments. I think of these guidelines as major landmarks for orientation on the movement landscape. Fortunately, they both point in the same basic direction.

RECOMMENDATIONS FROM HEALTH GROUPS

Numerous governmental agencies, including the World Health Organization, the U.S. Department of Health Services, and the National Health Service in the U.K., have published physical activity guidelines.[15] They are based on expert analysis of the voluminous research looking for correlations between physical activity, fitness and health. Here is a brief summary of their advice, which is almost the same for each source.

The amount

The guidelines suggest **at least** 150 minutes per week of "moderate" physical activity, or half as much "vigorous" activity. (See below for definitions.) The preferred amount of moderate activity is 300 minutes per week. Adding more exercise may continue to reduce mortality until as much as 750 minutes per week, after which point the health benefits of physical activity seem to flatline.[16]

"Moderate" activity defined

Moderate activities are usually light aerobic exercise — continuous cyclic movements done at an easy pace. Examples include:

- brisk walking
- hiking
- gardening or yard work
- jogging, cycling or swimming at an easy pace

Moderate exertion feels like you are working, but not in a way that is unpleasant or difficult to continue. Heart rate is about 60-80% of maximum, and breathing rate is elevated to a point where it would be difficult to sing, but easy to talk. You may break a light sweat but will not become significantly overheated. After finishing a session of moderate physical activity, you could probably complete another one if necessary.

"Vigorous" activity defined

Vigorous activity is higher intensity work that can be either continuous or intermittent. Examples include:

- resistance training with weights, machines, bands, or bodyweight
- sprinting or high intensity interval training on a cycle or rowing machine
- continuous running, cycling, swimming, or rowing at a challenging pace
- heavy manual labor

During continuous vigorous activity such as running or cycling, you are approaching the fastest pace you can sustain for twenty or more minutes. Your breathing rate is high enough that you cannot have a conversation. Intermittent activities like weight lifting, sports or sprinting cannot be performed continuously, but only in intervals. Vigorous physical activity feels hard and requires willpower to continue. When you are finished, you will probably want to rest at least a day before completing a similarly tough workout.

Movements that challenge strength

Most guidelines recommend that the above weekly totals should include at least two sessions that maintain or build strength in all major muscle groups. Although the majority of research on physical activity relates to aerobic exercise, there is a large and growing number of studies showing equally impressive health gains from strength training.[17] Some of these benefits are not available with aerobic exercise, especially preservation of muscle mass, which declines with age, often to a point where function is significantly compromised.

Movements that challenge mobility and basic coordination

Some popular guidelines, but not all, recommend inclusion of movements that maintain functional ranges of motion, and basic movement skills like squatting or single leg balance.[18] This doesn't mean you need exercises *specifically* devoted to this purpose, such as stretching or corrective exercise. Many common activities challenge mobility and functional movement skills, including dancing, swimming, martial arts, gymnastics, climbing, calisthenics, or classic compound strength exercises like pushups, pull-ups, rows, presses, squats and lunges. On the other hand, if all you do is bike or run, you will not be challenging your mobility or coordination very much.

PHYSICAL ACTIVITY LEVELS OF HUNTER-GATHERERS

Another way to approach the question of how to move is to consider the physical activity levels of humans living in more natural environments. This is the same logic you would apply to analyzing the health needs of any other animal. If you had a pet cheetah and wanted to know how much running she should do to maintain good health, you would try to learn something about how much cheetahs run in the wild. If you had a pet chimp, you would take him to the climbing gym, not the swimming pool.

Anthropologists who study hunter-gatherer cultures observe that they generally enjoy excellent health and fitness, and have low to non-existent rates of chronic diseases associated with a sedentary lifestyle.[19] They engage in high levels of physical activity, but certainly do not consider it to be exercise or medicine.[20] Movement is simply inseparable from almost every meaningful event in their lives. Although each hunter-gatherer culture has a different lifestyle, there are some general patterns and averages that are informative.[21]

Men usually spend the day hunting, which requires lots of walking, occasional jogging, and the odd sprint. They sometimes climb trees, dig to find tubers, and carry food back to camp, which must be butchered. Women generally spend their days gathering plants, and also caring for young children, who often must be carried. Back at camp, men and women engage in toolmaking, and food preparation. Down time is spent sitting on the ground in positions like squats that challenge lower body mobility.

Although they are moving all day, the pace is not grueling. Recent studies on the Hadza tribe in Tanzania show that they do about 135 minutes per day of moderate to vigorous physical activity.[22] That's about 900 minutes of activity a week, just a bit past the point at which recent studies have found that adding more exercise stops providing any significant additional health benefits in terms of reduced mortality.[23]

Some days involve hard work, but they are usually followed by easy days. Presumably some days will involve maximum intensity effort — sprinting, fighting, or carrying a heavy load. Interestingly, activity levels do not decline much with age. The 65-year-old elders keep up just fine with the young adults. A good percentage of the total workload is walking 5-10 miles per day.[24] If you think in terms of steps, this is about 10 to 20,000.

How does this organic, all-natural program for fitness compare to the standard issue government cheese? There are some obvious similarities. The majority of the work is moderate continuous movement like brisk walking. Vigorous activity is a smaller percentage of the whole, and includes work that challenges strength (climbing, digging, carrying, butchering) or power (sprinting). Many of the activities require mobility, coordination, and balance, such as walking over uneven terrain, climbing and scrambling, digging, lifting and carrying odd-shaped items, throwing, and sitting on the ground. One major difference is that hunter-gatherers do a higher volume of low intensity work, even compared to highly active modern humans. They are not doing more bench presses, but they are getting in far more steps.

Interestingly, walking is exactly the type of physical activity that modern humans would probably like to do quite a bit more, if only they had the time. Paddy Ekkekakis studies motivation to exercise, and observes that although high intensity exercise is quite effective at delivering health benefits quickly, most people don't do it because ... (prepare to be shocked) ... they don't like it.[25] But people tend to enjoy walking. Under the right circumstances, say being with a friend in a nice environment, they do not consider it to be exercise at all, but an enjoyable and invigorating experience that delivers immediate rewards.

Another notable feature of walking is that it provides health benefits with only a minimal risk of injury. More intense exercise (e.g., a set of barbell squats) offers a relatively narrow window between too much and not enough. The difference between a good workout and an injury might be just a few plates on the bar. But the margin of error with walking is huge. After a healthy dose of walking, most people could double it and recover easily.

It should not be surprising that walking is the healthiest form of physical activity, given this is the movement we are best adapted to perform. Like any other animal, our primary physical function is loco-motion, and walking is the most energetically efficient way to get the job done. If you did nothing else but walk a lot, you'd be in better shape than most Americans.

LOW-HANGING FRUITS

The diet analogy is informative not just for getting some ballpark aver-ages, but for finding the specific needs of a particular person. If you wanted the biggest payoff from eating a certain food, you would choose one that cures a nutritional deficiency. Limes are not often considered superfoods, but for people with scurvy, they are life-saving.

With exercise, working to improve a weakness would probably have more general benefit than improving a strength. If you can already run a six-minute mile, it won't be a life-changer to get your time down to 5:30. Also, it would be a lot of work to get there, and you would risk a repetitive stress injury along the way. But if you can't even do a cou-ple pushups, it would probably be pretty easy to get up to 10, and that might make a big difference in your overall functional ability. It's a low-hanging fruit.

This principle seems a bit obvious, but people ignore it frequently. In my practice, I see dancers who spend their spare time doing yoga, frail aging women who would never consider weight training, and buff football players who are only interested in their gym numbers. We have a tendency to train our strengths and ignore our weaknesses. This is understandable — part of what keeps us playing with movement is the internal reward that comes from a personal sense of mastery over physical tasks. But another aspect of play is the courage to try some-thing new without fear of failure. A playful attitude toward movement is one that doesn't worry too much about the embarrassments of doing something you're not good at. If you're willing to bear the shame of being an absolute novice for a little while, you might gain some capacities that make a real difference in your functional ability.

VARIABILITY OF PHYSICAL ACTIVITY

A healthy meal for one day is not a healthy meal *every* day. Similarly, a "meat and potatoes" exercise program (e.g., cardio, resistance training and stretching) is great. But when repeated in the exact same way for years, a change might be a good thing. This would rest areas that are repeatedly stressed, and direct work to some blind spots that are escaping challenge. Variability may also help avoid boredom. At the risk of using way too many food analogies, we should remember that variety is the "spice of life" in many areas, exercise included.

Good athletic coaches make sure to vary the training stimulus. You can't continue to make progress on the same program indefinitely. After a few months, returns will diminish, athletes will hit a plateau, and the workout will become stale and boring. Training should then be varied in some way that affords recovery from accumulated stress and stimulation of new adaptations.

There are many different ways to add variety to your physical activity, and each chapter of the book will hopefully provide some ideas, by looking at movement from different perspectives. One source of variation is manipulating the time and intensity of exercise. As noted above, popular guidelines offer some choices with these variables. "Vigorous" activity can provide similar benefits to "moderate" activity in only half the time.[26] You might be able to cut your workout even shorter with extremely high intensity work, done near maximum effort. For example, a commonly studied model for high intensity interval training is the use of 4-6 half-minute max effort sprints on a stationary bicycle, followed by four-minute recovery intervals at very slow pace. These improve certain health measures (e.g., cardiovascular fitness, skeletal muscle oxidative capacity and insulin sensitivity), as much as extended aerobic training.[27] In one study, participants completed just three reps of twenty-second max effort bicycle spirits, interspersed with two minutes of very low intensity cycling, three times per week for twelve weeks. They got similar results to another group working at moderate pace for 45 minutes per session.[28] Of course, the key here is that you really need to use a *max* effort, which many people may be reluctant to do. Further, it's unlikely that you can develop well-rounded fitness in just fifteen minutes per week. But including short, high-intensity workouts as an occasional change-up can make it easier to find time to exercise, add some unique benefits, and may even be fun. Personally, this kind of thinking has encouraged me to occasionally run around the block as fast as I can with the dog, or one of my daughters.

PLAYING WITH FITNESS

Here is my attempt to integrate and very briefly summarize the above information, using the central metaphor that runs through this book. If you want to "play" with fitness as a way to improve general health, here are some "rules of the game" to keep in mind. Have as much fun as possible within these basic constraints:

- Aim for at least half an hour and up to two hours of physical activity almost every day.
- Movement should be varied in terms of volume, intensity and type. Most activity can be fairly light. Walking is the most natural and beneficial movement for human beings.
- Occasionally include some high intensity work that significantly challenges your strength, power, and/or capacity to sustain high energy output for a short period of time. Climbing, running and resistance training are logical choices.
- Include movements that challenge coordination, balance, and range of motion.

Or to put this in even simpler terms:

- Move around a lot at a slow easy pace.
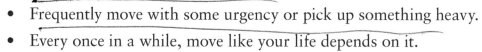
- Frequently move with some urgency or pick up something heavy.
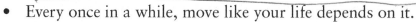
- Every once in a while, move like your life depends on it.

Here are a few notes and caveats to keep in mind.

First, these recommendations apply to a broad population. Obviously, everyone is different, and people need to explore many alternatives before finding what works best for them. A skilled trainer may significantly speed up the search based on your personal needs.

Second, consistency is more important than perfection. A suboptimal plan that is executed every week for years is way better than the perfect plan that is abandoned after a few weeks. Find a program that fits your schedule, abilities, social and environmental resources, and above all your personal interest and sense of meaning.

Third, something is far better than nothing. Physical activity is an essential nutrient with diminishing returns. If you are getting almost none, then adding just a little may provide a major payoff. The difference between nine and ten hours a week of exercise is negligible, but the difference between zero and one is huge.

Fourth, the guidelines are not specific directions. They are more like landmarks that you can use to stay oriented as you explore complex terrain. You should feel free to go down whatever pathways you find interesting. But every once in a while, make sure you aren't wandering through a desert.

Fifth, the guidelines are admittedly a bit reductionist. Although it can be useful to break down fitness into various component parts, this can lead to some bloodless exercise programs. Consider the typical gym-based exercise template: 5-10 minutes of stretching to address mobility; half an hour of stair mastering for aerobic endurance; 20 minutes of strength training on machines for all the major muscle groups. This is a comprehensive program for fitness that technically checks all the boxes. And for people who actually show up to do this workout on a regular basis, that's a wonderful thing. The problem is that when you divide physical activity into abstract component parts, so that they can all be precisely measured and accounted for, the result may be a workout that is disconnected from a sense of fun, spontaneity, community, natural environment, or meaning. If that is the cost of a workout that delivers the right percentages of all the RDA recommended nutrients, it may not be worth it! Do something that you enjoy doing and feels meaningful, even if it doesn't check every box in the guidelines.

6

ENVIRONMENT

When we try to pick out anything by itself,
we find it hitched to everything else in the universe.
—JOHN MUIR

Ask not what's inside your head,
but what your head's inside of.
—WILLIAM MACE

Cheetahs who live in zoos suffer from gastritis, kidney disease, high levels of stress and mortality, and low rates of mating.[1] You don't need to be a zoologist to see that most zoo animals just don't look happy. I recall watching a polar bear in New York's Central Park Zoo, swimming back and forth in his small pool. His underwater movements were hypnotically impressive, but after a few minutes I noticed he was repeating them over and over again in the exact same way without variation. He wasn't playing, he was stalking a prison cell.

Zookeepers know they can improve their animals' health by taking steps to "enrich" their physical and social environments. Enrichment encourages natural movement behaviors related to locomotion, climbing, hunting, or object manipulation. Cats like big fields, monkeys like trees, and they both enjoy playing with toys. I imagine the polar bear would have appreciated a bigger pool.

The modern environment for humans is a bit of a zoo as well, although far nicer in most respects, and usually with better Wi-Fi. Fortunately for us, we build our own cages, so we have a pretty good idea of how to keep them enriched. Of course, not everyone has the resources for as much enrichment as they might like. And even when we do, we don't always make the healthiest choices about what kinds of enrichments to purchase.

Most people are living in social and physical environments that don't encourage healthy movement. For example: a small apartment filled with digital screens; a neighborhood without safe or interesting places to walk; a long commute to work by car; a job that requires heavy computer work; social relationships that are maintained by smart phone and social media. Everything about this environment is telling you to stop moving and start sitting. These common conditions are a big part of the story of modern human movement health.

Social and environmental variables are key constraints on movement. They help set the conditions that either reward or punish us for being active or sedentary. Over time, our behavior will tend to fall in line with these incentive structures. We are all parts of larger systems, such as families, companies, and communities. If we find the wrong place in the larger scheme of things, we might feel like cogs in big wheels, ground down by forces outside our control. But if we are in a healthy environment — the right family, friends, jobs, neighborhood, walking path, yoga class, or soccer team — many pieces of the movement health puzzle fall into place effortlessly.

In this chapter we will discuss the social and environmental dimensions of movement health. This is a very big subject and we will only be scratching the surface here. It should also be noted that many of the relevant variables may not be under our control. If we live in a small cage, chances are we have to deal with it. Fortunately, part of what makes an enriched environment is the way we perceive it, and this is something we can change.

THE CONTEXT FOR MOVEMENT

My oldest daughter never did very much biking when she was in elementary school. If you asked her why, she would have said that biking is not one of her interests, or that she is just not the kind of person who likes to bike. In other words, she would have explained her biking behavior in reference to her internal psychological state. But this theory would not explain why, a few years ago on a camping trip, she spent almost all day biking for several days, seemingly enjoying every minute. She was on her bike within ten minutes of waking, and then on and off until ten minutes before going to bed. Why the sudden change? Did she have a transformative experience? Was she suddenly convinced that biking is actually a fun thing to do? No! Because as soon as she got home, she went right back to not riding her bike. The only thing that really changed on the camping trip was the environment. Her home environment for biking is actually not that bad — she has places to ride and friends to ride with. But the campsite was slightly more favorable — more space, less traffic, and perhaps most significantly, the absence of electronic devices! A small change in context caused a phase shift in her behavior.

Ecological psychology emphasizes the importance of context. The main premise is that humans are fully "embedded" in their environments, and therefore we can't understand them very well in the abstract. For example, movement always has some relationship to the outside world. Walking is about going somewhere — getting closer to one thing or further away from another. Movement always emerges from a constant back and forth between internal and external. We tend to underestimate the effect of the environment on our behavior, perhaps because we overestimate our self-control and agency.[2] We like to think we make choices based on internal psychological factors, such as knowledge, rationality, discipline or taste. For example, we play soccer because we are the kind of person who just likes to play soccer; we repeat sprint drills because we are disciplined; and we go to the gym because we have knowledge that exercise is healthy. And we don't do yoga, or dancing, or weightlifting because those activities just don't suit our taste. There's some truth to these ideas, but it is always *relative* to some external context, and the context is subject to change.

Over the years, my interest in playing different sports has shifted significantly, mostly based on who I'm playing with. I'm much better at racket sports than soccer, but I have put most of my recent efforts into soccer because my best friends are on the team. If my teammates were all jerks, I might have concluded that I don't really "like" soccer anymore. It's not always about the activity itself, but the social environment. If your friends are doing it, and you feel accepted and valued when doing it, you will probably enjoy doing it too. Why do people get so attached to CrossFit, Body Pump, or spin class? Part of what they like is the communal element and crowd energy.

Higher levels of physical activity are correlated with access to sidewalks and parks, and the walkability and aesthetic qualities of neighborhoods.[3] Social factors, including support from family and friends, predict adherence to exercise programs.[4] Dog owners walk twenty-two more minutes per day than cat owners.[5] They also bend over more often to pick up poop. Some disturbing research has shown that our memories of gym class correlate with physical activity level.[6] Were you traumatized playing dodgeball in PE? Chances are, you are spending less time playing team sports as an adult. Low socioeconomic status is associated with almost every bad health outcome you can imagine, including obesity and lower levels of physical activity. There is growing interest in the idea that certain diseases, including obesity, are in some sense "contagious."[7] A greater interest in exercise might also be something you can "catch" from friends.[8]

None of this means you need to buy some beachfront property or ditch your friends if they aren't fitness models or pro athletes. Despite the research showing the effect of social and environmental variables on physical activity, it remains the case that self-efficacy — the belief you can comply with an exercise program — is the best predictor of high levels of physical activity. You can go against the environmental grain if you are determined, but there is less friction in life when you go with it.

NATURAL ENVIRONMENTS

People like exercising outdoors better than indoors. It leads to higher levels of revitalization, cognitive attention, positive mood, and lower levels of anger, depression and tension.[9] As a result, people report a greater interest in adhering to "green exercise" programs. They also spontaneously select higher work rates when outside. For example, one study showed that during self-paced walking in natural environments, individuals walked faster, but reported lower levels of perceived exertion, compared to walking on a treadmill indoors.[10] In a similar study, exercisers were asked to maintain a given level of perceived exertion during cycling, and pedaled harder outside than inside, as reflected in higher speed, heart rate, and blood lactate concentration.[11]

One reason for this difference may be that movement through an outdoor environment provides sensory feedback that you are actually getting somewhere, which is the whole point of movement in the first place. It is likely that the body evolved mechanisms to conserve energy when physical activity isn't necessary, and this explains why most of us have an aversion to hard physical work that isn't compensated by some form of immediate payoff.[12] The visual perception of progress provides a feeling of reward that encourages more work.[13] In other words, as you pedal away on a stationary bike staring at the same wall, there is a part of you that can't help but notice that you aren't going anywhere. This leads to some questions, conscious or unconscious, about why all this effort should continue.

Another potential benefit of being outdoors is that it seems to facilitate social cohesion and interaction, which is another way to reduce stress and increase the reward value of exercise.[14] You will probably have a better conversation with your friend on a biking trip than sitting next to her on the next exercise bike at the gym. This makes the whole experience more enjoyable and less stressful.

Other research shows that exposure to nature can have benefits even when you're sitting still. Natural environments promote relaxation, stress reduction, immune system changes, better sleep, and faster healing times.[15] For example, hospital patients with a window looking into green space healed faster and requested less pain medication that those with a view of a brick wall.[16] Researchers have proposed that the benefits of natural exposure are not just about a good view, but smells, sounds, air quality, and the total experience of being outside.[17] We shouldn't get too romantic about the healing powers of nature, but science is starting to validate the idea that "forest bathing" is a good idea.

AFFORDANCES

James Gibson coined the term "affordance" to describe features of the environment that create possibilities for useful actions.[18] Classic examples of affordances are the handle on a tea cup, or the railing on a stairway. Each affords an easier way to perform a task. When affordances are perceived, they "invite" certain movement patterns. When we see a couch, we are invited to sit down. When kids see trees with low branches, they see the opportunity for climbing. Escalators afford the chance to ascend stairs without effort. Hiking trails invite exploration of physical space, while iPads do the same for virtual space. Thus, the presence of affordances will continually shape your movement behavior.

Some affordances are hard to detect even when they are right in front of your face. When a novice rock climber looks at a climbing route, he may not perceive the easiest pathway. But an experienced climber will immediately see the solution, e.g. the right foot moves to foothold A, at the same time that the left-hand leans on position B, which affords the possibility to reach a handhold at position C and so forth. Part of climbing skill is perceiving the hidden affordances that are there and ready to help you, if only you can see them. This is true in many other sports as well, especially team sports, where the relative positions of teammates, opponents, sidelines, and balls will determine movement opportunities. When Tom Brady drops back to pass, his eyes look on a rapidly changing landscape of opening and closing green spaces, with large men running left and right, colliding with each other, half of them trying to kill him. Most people would look at this scene and see only terrifying chaos, but Brady sees potential solutions: blockers he can hide behind, open spaces to run, receivers who can catch a pass. These affordances are hard to perceive because they are changing second by second. But Brady perceives them before they even arise.

A boxer is always watching his opponent to see whether his weight distribution, body position, and balance will afford him the possibility to move into position for a strike without exposure to a counterstrike. Top soccer players constantly scan the environment for movement possibilities afforded by the relative positions of teammates and opponents. The best players turn their head to search the environment once every two seconds.[19] All-time great soccer player Xavi from Barcelona explains how he does his job:

> Think quickly, look for spaces. That's what I do: look for spaces. All day. I'm always looking. All day, all day. Here? No. There? No. People who haven't played don't always realise how hard that is. Space, space, space. I think, the defender's here, play it there. I see the space and pass. That's what I do.[20]

Like a speed chess player, Xavi can read the field instantly and take effective action. This is why, as we will discuss in chapter ten, sport training or skill practice must include a representative environment. Decontextualized practice cannot train skill in perceiving affordances, which is fundamental to many sports.

AFFORDANCES IN THE MODERN WORLD

Modern environments are filled with affordances for sedentary behavior — comfy chairs, elevators, magical screens that help you explore the world with the swipe of a finger, and delicious foods within easy reach. One way to get moving is to eliminate some of these invitations to laziness. Katie Bowman removed couches from her living room to encourage more floor sitting, which challenges lower body mobility. Some similar environmental strategies to encourage healthy behavior would be keeping junk food out of sight, or hiding smartphones and laptops near bed time.

Home environments can also be enriched by adding things that invite more movement. I often leave soccer balls, kettlebells, or resistance bands in conspicuous areas of the house. Sometimes on purpose. I find pull-up bars especially attractive — I can't resist a few swings or hangs when I see that one is within reach. In my basement, I make sure to leave carpeted floor space free for rolling around or playing with my daughters. I was almost stupid enough to put a pool table in this space, which would have constantly invited me to spend hours every day with my chin over a cue stick. (I would have accepted.) Of course, there are many things about my home environment I can't change. I would love to have some nice hiking trails behind my house, but instead my back door opens onto a small patch of grass covered in dog poop. The reality is that most people are not in a position to make major changes to their environments. But perhaps they can change the way they see the environment.

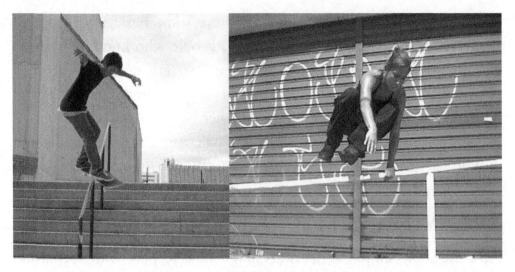

Figure 6.1. World as playground.

Skateboarding and parkour developed when people started to look at urban jungles as obstacle courses. By seeing the world in a different way, they invented new forms of movement. My friend Rafe Kelly started the first parkour gym here in Seattle.[21] The name of the gym, Parkour Visions, refers to the way parkourists see the world — benches are for vaulting, walls for mounting, poles for swinging. Different perception leads to different action. And this works in reverse as well — action changes perception. When you develop a new skill set, you see the opportunities to put it to use. What would happen if you developed some basic Parkour skills? You might start to see the world around you as a playground. When I learned rock climbing in graduate school, everything in my house started to look like a climbing wall. Me and my roommates were always traversing the moldings above the wide doorways. (We were idiots.)

I think this is a good reason to develop basic literacy in skills that can be used in the gym. For better or worse, fitness clubs are where many of us will find the most convenient and socially sanctioned opportunities for vigorous movement. I would be thrilled if my two girls continued their interest in playing outside and doing cartwheels into adulthood. The reality is that they will probably follow the social flow into gyms.

When they get there, I want them to have some basic knowledge of the territory and the skills to explore it. People who know how to do basic lifts like squats, deadlifts, and cleans are far more likely to look at a gym and see a playground. Not everyone will find gyms inspiring, but the success of CrossFit and many other box gyms was built on the reality that barbells, squat racks, gymnastic rings, medicine balls and pull-up bars can be *fun*. (They also fit pretty well into garages.)

PLAYING WITH THE ENVIRONMENT

Here are some simple suggestions about how to play with social and environmental constraints on movement health:

1. Put yourself into environments that encourage activity, especially outdoors. Enrich your indoor environment. Notice features of your surroundings that allow unique movement opportunities.

2. Develop basic literacy and appreciation for movements that can be done in *any* environment — walking, running, sprinting, jumping, climbing, throwing, dancing and gymnastics. You can't spontaneously cartwheel on a free patch of grass if you don't know how to cartwheel!

3. Explore movements that are well-suited to your current environment. If you live near a beach, learn how to swim and surf. If you live near the mountains, take up skiing and hiking. If you live near large football fields or tracks, train to improve your sprint time. If you have ready access to gyms, find out what kinds of exercises people really find meaningful or fun, and see if you can understand why.

4. Find social groups that encourage you to move, and that make you feel like a valued member of the group when you do. Avoid groups that make you feel guilty, ashamed, or incompetent. If you think you're just not the kind of person who likes a certain activity, ask yourself why. Do you hate dancing/dodgeball/lifting weights, or do you hate people judging you negatively for the

way you do these things? It is your solemn right to do things you suck at, especially when you're a novice. Find people who support you in what you want to do.

5. Take advantage of what the modern world has to offer. Although we are in some ways environmentally impoverished, we are in other ways amazingly enriched. With just a few internet searches, you can find instruction in martial arts, juggling, yoga, capoeira, soccer, kickball, gymnastics, javelin, and kayaking. If you want to learn a new dance step, there are hundreds of YouTube tutorials ready and waiting. No matter how weird your interest, there is an online community of like-minded people gathering information about it, analyzing it, sharing it, and most likely getting about half of it completely wrong. But they will share nuggets of wisdom and inspiration too. In an information age, the number of territories worth exploring has expanded exponentially. Not all are safe, but there's gold in them thar hills. For the curious, life is way too short.

7

STRUCTURE

The human body is the best picture of the human soul.
— *LUDWIG WITTGENSTEIN*

There is more wisdom in your body than
in your deepest philosophy.
—FRIEDRICH NIETZSCHE

The structure of the body — the muscles, bones, tendons, ligaments and connective tissues — is easily seen and measured. Because anatomy is right there ready to be MRI'd, foam-rolled, and scalpelled, people are quick to assume it's the key piece of the movement puzzle. This is especially true when the puzzle is pain, which is usually blamed on some form of structural damage, such as a bulging disc, torn rotator cuff, degenerative joint changes, or muscle knots. However, the correlation between tissue damage and pain is far weaker than you might imagine. Structure is overrated as a determinant of pain, and this leads to literally millions of unnecessary medical treatments.

On the other hand, structure is underrated in its effects on coordination. The shape of the bones helps determine what movements are most efficient and comfortable for a particular person. Because everyone has a different skeleton, they must explore to find what works best for them.

STRUCTURE AND FUNCTION

We all know you need to be big to be an NFL lineman, tall to play in the NBA, and small to be a jockey. But there are more subtle ways that structure affects movement.

Wingspan matters. Most people have arms that extend about two inches more than their height, but the average difference in the NBA is more than five inches. Kevin Durant is seven feet tall, but his arms extend to 7'5", which means his jump shot is almost impossible to block. Elite swimmers also benefit from long arms, which provide most of their forward propulsion. Michael Phelps is 6'4", and his wingspan is seven feet. But his legs are relatively short, about the same length as Hicham El Guerrouj, the world-record holder in the mile, who stands only 5'9". Phelps is all torso, Guerrouj mostly legs.

Hip joint structure affects athletic ability. Stu McGill, a leading biomechanics researcher, has noted that some hips are well-suited for powerful movement into flexion and extension, which helps you sprint in a straight line. Other hips are built more for lateral movement, which is a major asset in tennis or basketball.[1]

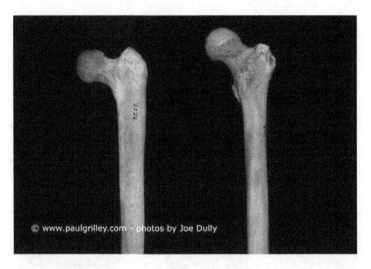

© www.paulgrilley.com - photos by Joe Dully

Fig. 7.1 The owners of these hips moved differently when they were alive.

Structure also matters for coordination. The intelligence that organizes movement is not just in the brain, but widely distributed all over the body, even in the shape of the bones. A well-designed structure can walk without assistance from a brain, or even muscles. Passive walkers are humanoid robots that walk with an eerily human gait, even though they don't have motors or computers. Do a YouTube search to see them in action. When they are put on a gentle slope and given a little push, they put one foot in front of the other. They remain upright because of the clever design of their skeletons. Human skeletons are also designed to walk, and this minimizes effort from the muscular and neural systems. Of course, some humans, owing to the shape and size of their skeletons, can walk and run far more efficiently than others. If you watch elite marathoners cruise along easily at speeds that most people can barely sprint, they might appear like a ball rolling downhill. Some people were just born to run. Others are born to throw a ball ninety miles an hour, or dance ballet.

Structure also impacts posture. In a scoliotic spine, the vertebrae and rib cage are asymmetrical, so a "neutral" position isn't straight. Asking someone with scoliosis to stand vertical is taking them out of a position which is the most efficient and comfortable for their structure.

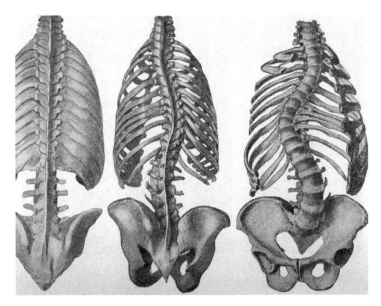

Figure 7.2: All three spines are in neutral.

Muscular structure has a huge impact on movement ability. Type I, or "slow twitch" muscle fibers, are metabolically efficient and perform well at moderate levels of work intensity for long periods of time. Type II, or "fast twitch" muscles, are far more powerful over short periods of time, but fatigue quickly. Most of us are about 50/50 in the ratio of fast to slow twitch muscle. But for some people the balance is far more lop-sided. Elite sprinters have a distribution that is closer to 70% in favor of fast twitch,[2] and marathoners are the opposite.[3] There is some debate about whether training can alter these percentages some small amount, but it appears that we are for the most part stuck with what our parents gave us.

Unlike many of the structural factors discussed above, the body's ratio of muscle to fat can be altered significantly in the short term. In certain contexts, this can have an immediate effect on coordination. Esther Thelen proved this by examining the effect of leg chubbiness on the stepping behavior of infants.[4] When tiny babies are held upright, they start stepping, as if they wanted to walk. As they get a little older, they stop stepping, and then start again a few months later. The prevailing theory to explain this was related to the nervous system — infants somehow acquire then lose the motor control programs required for stepping. But Thelen showed the cause was probably changes in the strength to weight ratio of the legs. Babies tend to stop stepping right at the same time their legs fatten up, and she got them stepping again by partially submerging their legs in water. This made the legs effectively lighter, and with this constraint changed, the system immediately reorganized. This should perhaps make us curious about how we would move differently after losing five pounds of fat, or gaining five pounds of muscle.

HOW STRUCTURE ADAPTS

The body's structure adapts to mechanical stress. When the stress exceeds a certain threshold, this initiates physiological changes that, if continued, will eventually make the stressed tissues better able to handle similar loads in the future. For example, when muscles are challenged by weight lifting, cells are damaged, and accumulate metabolic waste. Both of these conditions stimulate changes that promote muscle growth.[5]

Mechanotransduction is the process by which the cells of the body sense and respond to mechanical loads. Karim Khan describes mechanotransduction as:

> an ongoing physiological process in the human body, just like respiration and circulation. . . .[T]he process of regulating bone to load has been referred to as the "mechanostat." In the absence of activity, the mechanotransduction signal is weak, [causing] osteoporosis. When there are loads above the tissue's set point, there is a stimulus through mechanotransduction so that the body adapts by increasing protein synthesis and adding tissue where possible (larger, stronger bone).[6]

This shows that the hard structures of the body are more intelligent and adaptable than we might assume. Although they appear relatively static and senseless, bones, tendons and cartilage are always engaged, at the cellular level, in a dynamic process of trying to adapt to their conditions. Every day they grow slightly more or less capable of making certain movements safely. These adaptations may take months or even years to yield meaningful results, but they are ongoing.

Adaptations to structure are specific. For example, if you repeatedly contact a certain part of your heel during walking, this specific area of the heel will slowly grow larger and denser. It's a similar process to developing a callous on skin. Thus, the current structure of your body is the result of its "efforts," over many years, to adapt to the specific forms of mechanical and energetic stresses that it has experienced over its lifetime.

DAMAGE TO STRUCTURE

Many of my younger clients have told me they have been informed by a medical professional that they have the "knees of a fifty-year-old," or the "neck of an old man." These bogus diagnoses are often accompanied by a recommendation to stop doing a valued activity that might stress the supposedly infirm joints. This is usually horrible advice. If your joints feel good during and after healthy activities, the "age" of the joint is not a good reason to stop them.

It is true that as we get older, tendons dehydrate, discs bulge, injuries heal incompletely, and joint surfaces get rough. Many of these conditions result more from natural aging processes than specific pathologies. For example, degenerated discs are sometimes called "wrinkles on the inside" and they are probably due more to genes than environment.[7] But movement matters as well. Baseball players are more likely to have a torn rotator cuff in the throwing shoulder. Hockey can be hard on the hip joints. But these problems do not necessarily cause pain (see below), and they may be more about insufficient rest than excess movement. Repetitive stress will make tissues stronger if they have adequate time to recover.

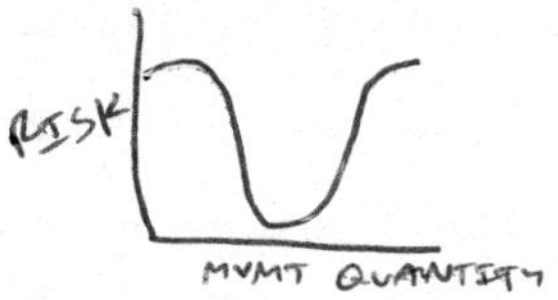

[handwritten annotation: RISK (curve) MVMT QUANTITY]

In fact, moving too little may be as bad for joints as moving too much. Running, which compresses discs, can make them stronger and healthier.[8] Although running stresses the knee, it does not increase the risk for knee osteoarthritis.[9] In fact, knee osteoarthritis increased dramatically after 1900, when people started moving *less*. One study showed that modern skeletons had 2.5 times more knee arthritis than their pre-industrial or prehistoric ancestors, who were far more active.[10] Thus, degenerative changes are not just about wear and tear, but rust. The healthiest amount of movement must somehow strike a balance between too much and too little.

Structural redundancy

In a machine, a local failure may cause a global catastrophe. The space shuttle exploded because of one defective O-ring. But living things are more robust than machines. They are built with structural redundancy, which allows them to perform the same function in many different ways.

Dogs who lose a leg can still move around with agility. In the Paralympics, people with missing limbs perform at the highest levels of intensity. There are many roads to Rome, and the body is designed to find them even when the most obvious pathways are blocked. At least nine different muscles can help flex the hip. If one is injured or fatigued, others take over. The same is true for almost any other basic movement in the body. The ACL is a key player in knee stability, but if it is torn, the hamstrings help pick up the slack. Many top athletes, including Mickey Mantle, Joe Namath and Thurman Thomas, played for years without a functional ACL. That doesn't mean it's a good idea, but it proves the body can be amazingly robust.

A case study in the British Medical Journal discusses a man who ran over twenty marathons, including a personal best in just over three hours, without a tibialis anterior muscle, one of the largest muscles in the lower leg.[11] The Canadian physical therapist and pain educator Neal Pearson tells a story about a retired NFL lineman who received cancer treatment that removed his psoas muscle.[12] The psoas runs right through the center of the body, and plays a key role in the gait cycle. It is sometimes suggested that even slight asymmetries in its function can discombobulate the whole body. What happened to the man who got one removed completely? He was running within six weeks of surgery, and later ran triathlons pain-free for ten years.

THE DISCONNECT BETWEEN STRUCTURAL DAMAGE AND PAIN

This section has a very important and optimistic message — structural damage to the body does not always cause pain, and pain is not always the result of structural damage. Confusion about these facts is the cause of a tremendous number of unnecessary and damaging medical treatments.

When a shoulder or knee starts to hurt, it is entirely normal to wonder whether tissue damage is causing the pain. So people will ask a doctor to order an MRI to have a look. Frequently, the MRI will show some form of damage, and the common thought process is that the cause for pain has been found, and surgical repair is the cure. This reasoning process is flawed, as revealed in two important lines of research. One is a series of studies showing that almost no matter where you point an MRI on a person over 30, you have a very strong chance of finding significant damage, *even in places without pain*. The second is research showing that many popular orthopedic surgeries to repair damage found on MRIs *work no better than placebo*. Following is a detailed review of the relevant research.

MRIS ON PEOPLE WITHOUT PAIN

In 1994, a study was done using MRIs to examine the backs of people without pain. It was discovered that about half had at least one bulging disc. The authors concluded that the presence of a bulging disc on someone with back pain "may frequently be coincidental."[13] In a similar study, it was found that one third of people without back pain had a substantial spinal abnormality, and 20% under the age of 60 had a herniated disc.[14] Pain-free necks look even worse under MRI. In a group of 1200 volunteers, 87% had bulging discs, including 76% of people in their twenties.[15]

In 2015, researchers collectively analyzed the results from 14 separate studies using MRI to examine the backs of people without pain.[16] They found that by age 30, about half have disc degeneration. By age 60, about a quarter have spondylolisthesis (when a vertebra slips significantly forward from another). By age 70, more than three quarters have a bulging disc. This is all for people without any pain. (See Figure 7.3 for more data.)

MRI Findings in Patients Without Back Pain By Age							
Image Finding	20	30	40	50	60	70	80
Disc degeneration	37%	52%	68%	80%	88%	93%	96%
Disc height loss	24%	34%	45%	56%	67%	76%	84%
Disc bulge	30%	40%	50%	60%	69%	77%	84%
Disc protrusion	29%	31%	33%	36%	38%	40%	43%
Annular fissure	19%	20%	22%	23%	25%	27%	29%
Facet degeneration	4%	9%	18%	32%	50%	69%	83%
Spondylolisthesis	3%	5%	8%	14%	23%	35%	50%

Figure 7.3: Happy backs often look sad under MRI. From Brinjikji (2015)

You may be thinking: "Okay, so these people aren't hurting right now, but what about in the future?" Several studies have addressed this issue. In one, a seven-year follow up found no correlation between initial MRIs and future pain.[17] Another study did a ten-year follow up, looking at the extent of disc degeneration, spondylolisthesis, disc bulge and other findings. The conclusion: "Our data suggest that baseline MRI findings cannot predict future low back pain."[18]

Similar studies have been done on hips, shoulders and knees. In a group of pain-free hockey players, 70% had abnormal pelvic or hip MRIs, and 54% had labral tears.[19] The author provided the following caution: "A surgeon may see something in the image, but it isn't causing a problem." In a study on asymptomatic knees in people aged 20-68, 60% had abnormalities, including meniscal tears.[20]

Researchers have found that the prevalence of rotator cuff tears in asymptomatic shoulders is "astonishingly high" — about 25% over age 50. They concluded that rotator cuff tears should be considered "normal degenerative attrition, not necessarily causing pain and functional impairment."[21] What about people using their shoulders for vigorous activity? In a group of pain-free overhead athletes, 40% of dominant shoulders had rotator cuff tears. These athletes remained pain-free five years after the study.[22]

Dr. James Andrews, a nationally recognized surgeon, scanned the shoulders of 31 healthy pain-free professional baseball pitchers, finding abnormal shoulder cartilage in 90 percent, and abnormal rotator cuff tendons in 87 percent. His conclusion: "If you want an excuse to operate on a pitcher's throwing shoulder, just get an MRI."[23] Andrews' concerns are reflected in new guidelines recommending against the use of MRIs in connection with recent onset back pain, which have been found to be associated with worse outcomes.[24] The cause for this association may include increased risk of unnecessary surgery, or reduced feelings of self-efficacy and optimism about recovery.[25]

Based on the above research, we know that tissue damage does not necessarily result in pain. *That doesn't mean it's irrelevant.* If you have a disc herniation or torn rotator cuff, pain is more likely. We can think of damage as kindling for a fire that may or may not be lit by other factors. See chapter eleven for more detail on what these factors might be.

MANY ORTHOPEDIC SURGERIES DON'T WORK

Unlike drugs, orthopedic surgeries can be sold to the public before they undergo rigorous testing to ensure they are safe and effective. Thus, millions of surgeries for knee, shoulder, and back pain have been done without studies to confirm they actually work. Recently, research has found that many popular surgeries (but not all) work no better than a placebo. And yet these surgeries are still done at the rate of hundreds of thousands per year. This is something you should know if you are considering surgery, or in the business of treating chronic pain.

Knee surgery

Osteoarthritis of the knee is common but does not necessarily result in pain — many people have arthritis and no pain at all.[26] But surgery to correct arthritis is popular, numbering as many as a half million per year in the U.S. alone.[27] About 15 years ago, two of the most common procedures were debridement (removal of damaged cartilage or bone) or lavage (irrigation with saline solution). The goal of either surgery was removal of rough fragments of cartilage that may be irritating the joint. The surgery's benefits were known to be not so impressive, so people started to wonder whether they were caused by placebo, or could be achieved with less invasive treatment.

To answer these questions, a study was done using a "sham" surgery: one group of patients received real knee surgery, and the other a fake, which involved just an incision on the skin. At several times over the course of a couple years, the two groups reported their levels of knee pain and function. The result? The sham group did just as well as the surgical group at all points in time.[28] This strongly suggests the surgery worked by changing psychology, not structure.

This study was slow to have an effect on the behavior of surgeons. Years later, hundreds of thousands of these surgeries were still being performed at the cost of $3 billion a year.[29] Subsequent research confirmed they provide no more benefit than common sense interventions like exercise, weight loss, and the occasional use of over-the-counter pain medicine.[30] Debridement and lavage eventually became less common, but were soon replaced by arthroscopic partial meniscectomy. But the new surgery proved to be equally weak. Like its predecessors, it worked no better than a sham. In 2015, researchers summarized the results of nine studies on arthroscopic procedures for the knee, and concluded they showed little if any benefit, and the possibility for serious harm.[31] Further studies in 2017 came to similar conclusions.[32]

A recent editorial in the *British Journal of Medicine* offered the scathing opinion that arthroscopic surgery for knee pain is: "a highly questionable practice without supporting evidence of even moderate quality."[33] A 2017 clinical guideline made a "strong recommendation against the use of arthroscopy in nearly all patients with degenerative knee disease" and noted that "further research is unlikely to alter this recommendation."[34] In spite of this advice, arthroscopic knee surgery continues to be the most common orthopedic procedure in the U.S., with close to 700,000 performed each year.[35]

Why the disconnect between research and practice? The simple answer is that many doctors trust their personal experience over controlled research. They will say they have seen surgery provide benefit after conservative therapies failed. Surely this sometimes occurs, but we should be skeptical that the cause is structural change in the knee. Instead, successful treatment for chronic knee pain, through surgery or otherwise, may be caused by complex changes in psychological or neurological processes.

Back surgery

Several back surgeries perform no better than conservative care. For example, vertebroplasty injects bone cement into fractured vertebrae. A study published in 2003 showed it works as well as no treatment at all after six weeks.[36] In 2009, two studies showed it worked no better than a sham procedure for fractures related to osteoporosis.[37]

Low back fusion is intended to enhance low back stability. In 2013, the *Spine Journal* published a study comparing spinal fusion to non-operative treatment, such as cognitive behavioral therapy and exercise. It found no difference in long-term outcomes, and concluded that "the use of lumbar fusion in chronic low back pain patients should not be favored" over conservative care and exercise.[38] In 2014, an analysis of multiple studies concluded that:

> There is strong evidence that lumbar fusion is not more effective than conservative treatment in reducing perceived disability because of chronic low back pain among patients with degenerative spinal diseases.[39]

As with knee surgery, research has been slow to affect practice. Nikolai Bogduk, an internationally renowned anatomist and back pain expert, explains that:

> Surgeons and others believe that surgery is effective for back pain. They base this belief either on their own experience or on observational studies. This belief is, by and large, not vindicated by the outcomes in well-reported clinical trials. Those trials indicate that only a small proportion of patients do well from surgery.[40]

Shoulder surgery

The research on shoulder surgery is less clear, but recent studies reveal a similar pattern. As noted above, pain-free shoulders often have torn rotator cuffs. Despite this fact, the most common diagnosis for shoulder pain is "impingement" of the rotator cuff by the acromion process, which is directly above.

Surgeries to correct these conditions include rotator cuff repair, or acromioplasty, where a portion of the acromion is removed. In the United States, there are almost half a million of these surgeries performed each year, most of them on shoulders where the damage is degenerative (caused by wear and tear and aging) as opposed to traumatic (caused by acute injury).[41] Are these surgeries more effective than exercise or rest? The evidence is less clear than with backs and knees, but it raises questions about whether the good results are caused by mechanical change in the shoulder. Although we cannot rule out the possibility that surgery will be substantially more effective than exercise for certain patients,[42] several studies have found that popular shoulder surgeries, such as acromioplasty, are no better than exercise.[43] Further, it has been shown that labral repair and biceps tenodesis surgeries do not outperform sham surgery.[44]

There is also evidence suggesting that even when surgery is effective at relieving pain, this is not because of structural repair.[45] MRIs of repaired rotator cuffs taken within a year after surgery often show that the cuff has fallen apart again, even though the patient has recovered.[46] A 2017 study compared two kinds of shoulder arthroscopic surgery (with and without decompression), and found that neither provided a clinically significant benefit over no treatment at all.[47] An editorial said these findings "send a strong message that the burden of proof now rests on those who wish to defend the standpoint that shoulder arthroscopy is more effective than non-surgical interventions."[48]

None of the above means that we should not trust orthopedic surgeons, or that surgery should never be used to treat chronic pain. Many surgeries have been proven to work, and are definitely a good idea under certain circumstances. I personally know many people who have received ethical advice from their surgeons, and got dramatic benefits from surgery. I also know people who got a surgery that had been proven to be ineffective, were never advised of the relevant research, and ultimately did not get a good result.

I think the lesson here is that the medical establishment has some biases in the way it treats chronic pain. It favors treatments based on simple structural explanations for pain, and tends to ignore complex neurophysiological processes that may be more important. We need to be aware of these biases and learn as much as possible about the complexity of pain so that treatment can be improved. And chronic pain clients need to ask their surgeons some good questions before going under the knife.

STRUCTURE AND MANUAL THERAPY

Physical therapists, massage therapists, and chiropractors generally consider their view of the body to be far less reductionist than that of an orthopedic surgeon. However, many of their pain treatment methods are similarly focused on structure. Popular techniques like spinal manipulation or myofascial release are premised on the alleged ability of the therapist to make significant and meaningful changes to hard structures — bones, muscles and fascia — in just minutes, using nothing more than hands! Although these therapies can sometimes help with pain, it is unlikely that this is caused by meaningful changes to the targeted structures.

Fascia doesn't "melt"

"Myofascial release" is a manual therapy technique sometimes advertised as a way to modify the length or tension of fascia, through use of mechanical forces applied by hands, metal instruments, or foam rollers. The rationale is that mobility can be improved if fascial adhesions or scar tissues are broken up or "melted."

This story seems to fail some basic tests of common sense. Wouldn't melting an important body part constitute a severe injury? If a therapist's hands can break parts of your body, shouldn't you fear them? And why would the connective tissues in the body, which are presumably organized in a highly adaptive manner, start to fall apart whenever they receive some sustained pressure? That would be surprising. Indeed, research shows that the pressure required to deform mature fascia is beyond what can be applied with hands, foam rollers or even steel tools.[49] We aren't made of clay. If we were, our backsides would be misshapen after sitting for few minutes on a park bench. Although myofascial techniques have been shown to increase flexibility and reduce pain, the mechanism probably involves changing neurophysiological processes related to perception or coordination, not structure.[50]

Bones don't snap "in" and "out" of place

Some chiropractors advertise the ability to change the alignment of bones, especially the vertebrae. The claim is that they can identify joints that are "out" and then crack them back "in" with an adjustment, which is also called spinal manipulation. Although bones can certainly move at their joints, it is quite another thing for them to snap in and out of place like pieces of plastic in a children's toy. When a joint violently pops from one place to another, as opposed to moving smoothly through a normal range of motion, this usually indicates an injury or dislocation, not a beneficial realignment.

The popping sound created by a chiropractors' adjustment is called a cavitation, and is probably caused by a small movement of the vertebrae away from each other and then back together.[51] There is no evidence that cavitations create meaningful long-term repositioning of the vertebrae, and studies have shown that manipulation cannot change the position of the sacroiliac joint or the neck.[52] More importantly, chiropractors are not able to predict *which* vertebrae will cavitate on a given manipulation.[53] That is likely because the forces created by a manipulation are distributed over a broad area, and cannot be targeted to a specific location.[54] In any event, the efficacy of an adjustment does not seem to depend on whether a cavitation occurs.[55] Further, simply mobilizing a joint provides a similar benefit to cracking it, as does mobilizing vertebrae at random, compared to selecting a specific vertebrae that is supposedly out of place.[56] Although spinal adjustments can relieve pain and improve range of motion, the likely mechanism is once again complex and neurophysiological, not simple and structural.[57]

Muscles don't have "knots"

Another misconception is that "muscle knots" are a common cause of pain or stiffness.[58] To be fair, no one actually believes that muscles can literally get tied into knots. But people do think they can contract into a palpable ball, that the ball is the cause for pain, and that some kind of deep pressure is required to "get in there" and release the tension.

Some classic areas where people complain of knots are the upper traps, or between the shoulder blades. There is no doubt muscles in these areas can feel tight and sore after activities where they are used for long periods of time, such as working at a computer. And pain may be related to associated muscle fatigue. But the subjective *feeling* of tightness is not the same as actual mechanical tightness. In fact, it is unlikely that stressed muscles become palpably tight. Studies looking for abnormal levels of EMG activity in relaxed but sore muscles are mixed, and others show that skilled massage therapists are unable to palpate a client's back and predict which areas feel tight to the client.[59] Other research shows that painful areas in the upper traps are actually less tight (as measured by an algometer) than surrounding areas![60] So next time you feel what you think is a hard area in a muscle, check whether it lies directly over a vertebra or rib. In my experience, most "knots" are sharp bones under thin slips of muscle.

PLAYING WITH STRUCTURE

We might summarize the foregoing by noting that structure is generally overrated as a constraint on how we feel, and underrated (in some ways) as a constraint on how we move. That being said, we should now ask: what are the constraints on structure that we might hope to modify, and thereby improve movement health? Some of the important variables are outside our control. No one is going to get taller by hanging from a bar, Bobby Brady style. But over long periods of time, the body has an amazing ability to adapt.

Here's a remarkable example to illustrate. A rare condition causes some children to be born without a tibia, which is the larger of the two bones in the lower leg.[61]

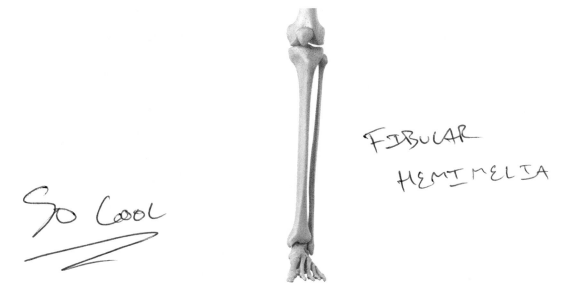

Figure 7.4: A normal lower leg with both tibia and fibula.

One treatment for this condition is to surgically relocate the fibula to where the tibia should be, directly under the knee. The fibula now has to deal with the mechanical stress of bearing weight, and in just a few years this transforms the fibula into a bone that looks just like a tibia! (To see a before and after picture, do a google image search for "fibula becomes tibia.") It's an amazing example of adaptation and self-organization. We tend to think that bone shape is determined by genetic code, but in this case the more important constraint is environmental. Of course, these extreme adaptations are only possible when you are very young, and the body is still highly plastic. During the time your structural foundation is being built, there is plenty of opportunity to make alterations in the basic layout. But once the house has been framed, there is far less in the construction budget to rip everything down, tear it out and start over.

Although adults cannot make major changes to the shape of their skeletons, they can make dramatic body transformations by adding muscle and/or losing fat. How much can we expect these changes to improve function? It depends on what you're doing of course. Dropping twenty pounds of fat will certainly make you a better runner, just as adding it will improve your performance in sumo wrestling.

Strength training and greater muscle mass will protect you from injury during sport and probably assist power generation in sports where power is needed, like baseball or football.[62] But the idea that larger muscles equals more power is less certain than you might imagine. For example, sprinters obviously benefit from high levels of strength and muscularity, and these factors are clearly correlated with elite performance. Further, there is significant research showing that resistance training can improve sprint times. But sprinting is also improved by, well . . . sprinting, and you have more time and energy for sprinting if you aren't doing heavy squats. Carl Lewis, one of the greatest sprinters in the history of the sport, had already won eight gold medals before he hit any weights at all, and started with numbers that would not impress the average gym bro.[63]

Long-distance runners seem to benefit from a little bit of strength training, but the effects are small, and probably unrelated to increased muscular size.[64] Runners want to be as light as possible, so small size, especially in the lower leg, is associated with better performance.[65] Thus, although middle distance runner Mo Farah credits his double gold in the 2012 Olympics to the addition of some strength work in his training regimen, we are not talking about any major weightlifting. Prior to training, Farah could barely do a pushup, and he was at that time number one in the world at his sport.[66]

For the most part, the best way to develop the structural adaptations that will assist your performance in a particular activity is to . . .

do that activity. Work at some level that you can easily tolerate, and then slowly progress over time. That's the SAID principle. The body specifically adapts to imposed demand. Even when armed with a tremendous amount of specialized know-how, it is hard to improve on this plan for optimizing the status of your structure for a particular purpose. Training off the field certainly provides important benefits in terms of performance and injury protection, but is always more of a supplement than the main course.

MOBILITY

With freedom comes responsibility.
— ELEANOR ROOSEVELT

Mobility means how well you move near a functional end range of motion. This is a slightly different concept from flexibility, which is more about *quantity* of motion than *quality*. For example, if two people squat to the same depth, they have the same flexibility in the ankle, hip and knee. But they might have different mobility: one moves to end range with speed, strength, balance, and control, while the other gets there slowly, with stiffness, weakness, or discomfort. So flexibility is about the length of the road: how far does it go before it hits a dead end? And mobility is more about the quality of the road at your intended destination. How wide are the streets, what is the speed limit, are there potholes or traffic jams? And is there good parking?

In most sports, mobility is probably the more important constraint on performance and injury prevention. Athletes usually don't require extreme ranges of motion, but rather extreme control at the end of relatively normal ranges of motion. For example, the hip muscles of a football

133

running back don't need to stretch that far — you won't see them doing the splits to avoid a tackler. But they perform incredibly challenging tasks in extended positions — decelerating, balancing, stabilizing, handling loads, and getting prepared to explode in the opposite direction.

MODELS OF FUNCTIONAL MOBILITY

A sprinting cheetah is a good model of functional mobility. As it chases dinner at high speed, its spine moves through large but controlled ranges of motion. The back rounds into flexion as the front and back legs come together, and then arches into extension as the legs reach apart. Although the middle spine is highly mobile, the upper back and neck maintain a steady head position, so the eyes stay locked on the target, like a camera on a moving dolly.

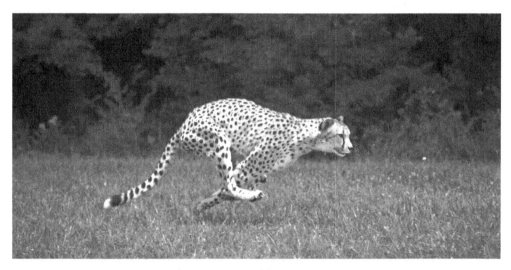

Figure 8.1. Fluid movement.

This coordinated movement requires the right level of mobility. The joints need to be loose enough to achieve the necessary ranges of motion, but not so loose as to be floppy. When the musculoskeletal system has too much slack, it is less connected, responsive and controllable. Joints move out of position and cause damage. So we need freedom of movement, but not so much freedom to allow chaos.

Many different constraints keep the body attracted to an optimal balance of flexibility and stiffness. The bones create hard barriers against unwanted movement, while discs, joint capsules and ligaments provide some "give" that allows small amounts of "play" in the joints. Tendons and connective tissues also limit range of motion, but only after a bit of stretch. The stretch creates elastic recoil that can be used to power movement in the opposite direction. Muscles control motion in a highly variable way, because they can relax or contract at the command of the nervous system. And the nervous system makes its decisions based on perceptions about how to achieve functional goals, and protect the body in the process.

The precise settings of all these different governors on mobility is differentiated, finely tuned, and adaptable. For example, a strip of connective tissue might stretch easily at one angle, but provide stiff resistance to movement at a slightly different angle. Over time, it will slowly adapt its structure to allow movement where needed, aligning its fibers with habitual lines of pull. A tendon can remodel to be stiffer and stronger, and these structural changes might take many months. The nervous system can change in an instant. It constantly modifies the length or stiffness of muscles, based on how it perceives needs for safety and function.

How do the cheetahs train up all these different constraints on mobility to ensure optimal performance? Of course, you won't see them doing anything that looks like a deliberate effort to stay limber, aside from a quick stretch after a nap. They certainly aren't foam rolling or getting deep tissue massages. Their lifestyle provides all the inputs needed to ensure the system will self-organize in an adaptive way, bringing into balance a whole orchestra of different variables that create functional movement.

Most modern humans follow the cheetah's "plan" for mobility development, at least for a while. From infancy until age six or seven, a child's mobility is shaped mostly by unstructured play, and the results seem to be pretty good. If you watch elementary school kids move, you will notice that most have the range of motion to perform the following movements with ease, many of which would trouble a middle-aged adult:

- Sit comfortably on the ground for extended periods of time in many different positions, including cross-legged, with extended legs, kneeling, or in a deep squat;
- Move to and from the ground in various squat and lunges patterns, with the feet in a variety of positions, including close together, far apart, staggered, on the toes, or flat-footed;
- Lift a foot to waist level at various angles to step onto an elevated surface or to deliver a kick;
- Fully extend an arm overhead at various angles to grab an object or hang from an overhead support, such as a bar or tree branch;
- Bend or rotate the spine as necessary to allow all the above movements and more, including crawling, climbing, jumping, running, falling, tumbling and rolling.

All these movements can be done at speed and under moderate levels of load. Although kids are flexible in these common movements, they are by no means contortionists. Many struggle to reach past their toes in a forward bend, or to emulate even simple yoga poses. But they have the mobility to do what healthy kids want to do: run, climb, sit, throw, kick, fall, dance, roughhouse, play sports, etc.

USING IT OR LOSING IT

As kids age, they tend to slowly lose their freedom of movement. By college, most will not be comfortable sitting for an extended time in a deep squat (assuming they can get into this position at all). Their movements up and down from the floor will probably have less variability and smoothness. By age 30, aggressive dance moves or karate kicks are inhibited by the fear of hamstring or groin injuries. At 40, some people have difficulty getting the arms fully extended overhead, especially at speed or in combination with arching and rotating the upper back.

But it would be a mistake to think losing mobility is mostly about getting older (although that certainly doesn't help!). Like many other qualities of movement health, mobility is relatively easy to preserve so long as it is used at some minimum frequency. For example, people who habitually sit in deep squats, as is common in certain Asian countries, and every hunter-gatherer culture, retain their ability to do so well into old age. I recall walking through the streets of Vietnam and seeing 80-year-old men and women eating soup or waiting for a bus while sitting on their heels. Even more impressive was their ability to move smoothly back and forth into this position from standing.

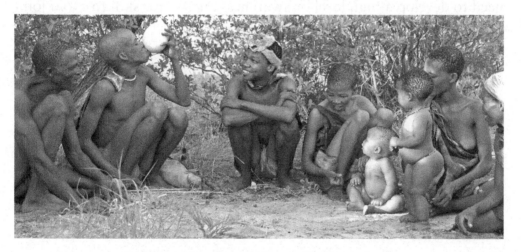

Figure 8.2. Hunter-gatherers in the living room.

In Western cultures, we spend lots of time in chairs or couches, and very little on the floor. We don't often use the end range of motion in the ankles, knees, and hips, so we lose it over time. A similar pattern occurs in the upper body, but more slowly. As we age, we reach more for the computer mouse or remote control, and less for tree branches and monkey bars.

Thus, the mobility system seems to be organized around the principle of use it or lose it. Babies are born with all the mobility they need and much more to spare. The bones at their joints are well spaced, and the tissues holding them together are soft. As time goes by, they gradually get rid of the flexibility they don't use. This is a good thing, because flexibility has a price. People with genetic connective tissue disorders such as Marfan's syndrome or Ehlers Danlos have very flexible tissues, and this makes them hypermobile. Their elbow and knee joints hyperextend, they can bend forward to put their palms on the floor with ease, and their skin is conspicuously stretchy.[1] This allows them to perform amazing feats on the dance floor or in the circus tent, but also increases the risk for joint damage and chronic pain. Further, hypermobility places more demand on coordination. When movement isn't constrained by structure, the nervous system needs to work harder to provide control. In some extreme cases, people with hypermobile joints need to develop a high level of awareness and motor skill to avoid joint dislocations in everyday movements.

Another cost of floppy joints is loss of efficiency and power. Just as a golf ball will bounce higher than a deflated tennis ball, a tight muscle or tendon has more spring. This is why elite runners have stiff hamstrings and ankles, and relatively poor range of motion into a forward bend.[2] They use their stiffness to bounce down the road. So there are tradeoffs with mobility. It's good for some things and bad for others, and the body will tend to get rid of any movement slack it doesn't need.

MOBILITY AND INJURY

It is commonly believed that working to improve flexibility is a good way to prevent injury in sport. The logic is that many injuries, especially muscle pulls, occur by exceeding the safe range of motion, and therefore increasing that range might create a protective buffer zone. This is one reason athletes stretch hamstrings and adductors. However, research is mixed on whether flexibility in either muscle group is correlated with injury risk.[3] More importantly, stretching programs have shown only limited efficacy in reducing muscle pulls.[4] This is consistent with a large body of research on stretching in general, which has failed to produce evidence showing any benefit in reducing sport injury.[5]

What seems to work better in preventing hamstring and groin injuries is strengthening, especially eccentric exercise, which occurs when the muscle is working to prevent further lengthening. For example, the Nordic hamstring exercise[6], and the Copenhagen adductor exercise[7], which both improve eccentric strength in the target muscles, are effective in reducing hamstring or groin injuries in athletes.[8] These findings make sense in light of the logic discussed earlier. The risk of moving a joint to end range is failing to control continued movement in the same direction. Strength training, especially near end range, challenges and builds the capacity to slow continued lengthening, handle heavy loads, and reverse direction. Thus, the best way to prevent injury is not so much about lengthening the road, but improving your ability to slam on the brakes and shift into reverse. Learning to control the steering wheel, through challenges to coordination and balance at end range, is not a bad idea either.

PLAYING WITH MOBILITY

Functional range of motion is relatively easy to maintain. Animal studies have shown that joints immobilized into shortened positions do not lose range of motion if they are extended for as little as fifteen minutes per day.[9] So you don't need to worry about your joints slowly knitting themselves together if you are not constantly mobilizing and stretching. Cats sleep 20 hours, wake up, have a quick stretch, and then . . . move like cats. They maintain their mobility by engaging in basic functional activities at some minimum frequency.

What are some basic functional activities that will maintain a healthy level of general mobility in humans? One way to answer this question is to look at the movements all healthy kids do spontaneously on a playground. Climbing, hanging, and swinging from monkey bars will challenge the shoulders to push and pull at every conceivable angle.

Every joint in the lower body gets a multi-planar mobility test by moving to and from the ground in variable patterns of squats and lunges. These specific activities are not *necessary* to maintain mobility, but they are probably sufficient. In fact, just climbing would keep you very mobile, even if that's all you ever did. Imagine being on a climbing structure with many potential hand and foot holds. You could very easily test every functional range of motion you have, simply by reaching for distant points in all directions with a hand or foot. Try this for ten minutes and see if anything feels left out.

You don't need a climbing wall to use this same basic template for playing with mobility. Get into any position that is functional for a wide variety of activities — standing, squatting, all fours, lunging, sitting in various positions on the floor. Now reach a hand (or foot) to a random distant point on the floor or the air, while keeping your other points of contact with the floor. (Yes, this is basically the game of Twister.) For example, get into a bear crawling position – feet flat on the ground in a squat position, hands palm down in front of the feet. Now lift the right hand and reach for as many different points on the floor as you can, as if you were painting a large circle with your hand. For a harder test, reach the hand to imaginary targets in the air so you paint a sphere. What muscles groups are stretching here? Something in the hips, trunk or shoulder? Yes.

For an easier set of movements, try the same thing while sitting in a chair, reaching the right hand as far as possible down and up, front and back, left and right. Make sure to really reach to an imaginary target, as if each millimeter counts, while keeping at least some part of your pelvis on the chair, or your feet anchored to the floor. This will cause you to include distant parts of the body in the movement, so the ribs and pelvis work with the shoulder. Depending on where you reach, your pelvis and spine will flex, extend, side-bend, and rotate. Explore all the different possibilities and what they feel like, noting that many will feel like functional, real-world movements. Repeat the ones that feel good or useful, adding in subtle variations in angle, posture, speed, etc.

Why does reaching to random points lead to movements that feel coordinated and familiar? Our primate ancestors lived in trees and spent a lot of time reaching for tree branches in random locations. Our bodies are well-organized to serve the needs of the hands to grasp distant things, and therefore reaching tends to get the body coordinated, especially into lengthened positions. When you reach, the body gets long in an intelligent way.

Feet can be used for reaching, especially in climbing. You can play with reaching the foot in a standing position, and easily test all your potential ranges of motion in the hip. Try reaching a foot to touch various points on the wall, while facing toward, away, and sideways from the target. Use the hands as much as you want for balance. If you reach the foot away from you along the floor, you will come into various lunge positions. This ends up being a strength workout for the supporting leg, showing that some forms of mobility are really about stability. You can get the same effect with the arms in push-up position, sliding one hand forward along the floor while the other works to prevent you from falling.

The sit bones can "reach" as well. Part of their function is to make contact with surfaces that afford sitting, so reaching them toward a chair will create natural movements. Try lowering your butt to an adjustable stool. Easy? Move the seat lower, further away, or to the left or right. Use different foot placements — close together and wide apart, heels up or down, and include asymmetry. Try to touch one sit bone but not the other. You can use this simple game to explore the entire landscape of squatting possibilities. You can explore lunging by getting into a staggered stance and reaching your back knee to the ground, or your front hand to points in front of you.

As we will discuss in chapter ten, the body coordinates itself best when attention is directed to some external goal in the environment. Internal attention will tend to make your movements stiff and awkward. Therefore, to play with mobility effectively, think in terms of reaching a target, not lengthening individual muscles or mobilizing joints. If you reach for a wide variety of targets from different postures, you will go a long way towards developing good general mobility, without consulting anatomy charts, making lists of muscles and joints to stretch, or engaging in arbitrary and non-functional movements like sitting with the feet together and pushing the knees down to stretch the groin.

What if you reach and come up way short of your goal? Maybe you have lost significant range of motion at a particular joint through disuse or injury. Prevention is easier than cure for most things, mobility included. So if for some reason you lose flexibility, restoring it might require a methodical approach that looks more like work than a game of Twister. The first step might be finding out what is limiting range of motion.

If flexibility is limited by the skeleton, there's not much you can do to improve it. Elbow extension is limited by the bones in the elbow joint, not the flexibility of the bicep. Other examples where motion is often constrained by the bones are big toe flexion, ankle dorsiflexion, hip flexion (with bent knees), and shoulder flexion. Several of these joint motions are involved in squatting. Some people can squat all the way down to the ground while maintaining a neutral curve in the low back. Others will find that the pelvis rolls under before the thighs reach parallel. The difference may be in the shape of the hip joint. A shallow hip socket provides more range of motion (but less stability), while a deep socket provides more stability and less range. Dancers have hip joints that are very well-suited for large ranges of motion in all directions. A study of approximately 50 male and female ballet dancers found that close to 90% had borderline dysplasia, a condition that affects only 1-5% of the general population.[10]

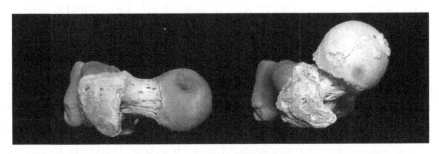

Figure 8.3: Top down view of two femurs: same knee position,
very different hip rotation.

Other features of the hip affect mobility. Figure 8.3 shows two femoral heads rotated at very different angles, even though each knee is facing forward. One of these people would be very good at rotating the hip out, the other inward. I have almost no internal rotation in my hips at all, and the limitation is probably bony not muscular. I can tell because of the "end feel" of the movement. The motion stops abruptly without any sense of stretch in the surrounding muscles, therefore the barrier is probably in the joint not the muscles. This is what it feels like when you fully extend the elbow. Compare that to a forward bend, or the splits, where you feel it in the hamstrings or adductors. If you are trying to get more range of motion and feel most of the stress in the joint and not the muscle, you may be asking for trouble.

The nervous system also constrains range of motion. If it perceives threat related to a muscle lengthening, it will stiffen the muscle to protect the body. Imagine you are standing on ice and feel your feet slip apart, taking you into the splits. You will reflexively tighten the adductor muscles to prevent a groin tear. Perception of threat makes you stiff. In a more relaxed environment — say a yoga class where you are sitting on the floor, in full control of your body, and otherwise completely chilled out — your nervous system will allow the adductors to relax into greater length. Each time you practice a stretch without excess discomfort, you are helping to "convince" the nervous system that the stretch is safe. In fact, "stretch tolerance" is probably the mechanism by which most stretching programs serve to increase flexibility.[11]

If threat reduction is indeed a pathway toward better mobility, we would expect that pain would be counterproductive. Indeed, experimentally induced pain has been shown to reduce flexibility.[12] And getting rid of it completely can lead to dramatic improvements. A recent study on people with "frozen shoulder" found that most of them immediately regained almost full range of motion after receiving anesthesia.[13]

This should get us thinking about the best ways to convince the nervous system that reaching a particular range of motion is safe. We would expect that extreme ranges of motion are best achieved by moving slowly, under control, and with a relaxed mind state. In other words, something like a yoga class. What if you need to move into an end range of motion with speed, power, balance, and under load? Then you need to start challenging your body to do exactly those things, starting with the easiest and least threatening movements (static, stable, slow, low force), and then gradually progressing the level of the challenge (dynamic, unstable, fast, with high force). I think of improving mobility as slowly retaking territory that has been lost. Go as far as you can safely, establish some confidence and functionality at that range, and then try to go further next time. As noted earlier, developing strength at the frontier may be especially helpful. Regardless of the exact mechanism, the solution to getting more flexibility or mobility is relatively simple — challenge the body to handle load and perform functional activities at the end range of motion, and it will adapt in multiple ways (e.g. structurally and neurologically) to get better at doing that.

9

POSTURE

Trying to move without good posture is like trying to write with a floppy pencil.
—NICOLAI BERNSTEIN

Sit up straight.
—POSTURE POLICE

What is good posture? To answer that question, we need to know what posture is *for*. The purpose of good trunk and neck alignment[1] is not to create an appearance of verticality or upstandingness to a critical observer. It is to help you efficiently and safely accomplish some physical task, such as standing, sitting, walking, running, reaching, etc. So posture should be judged by how you perform and feel, not by how you look.

The most fundamental function of posture is getting the head into a position that keeps you balanced and able to see the world around you. Head control is one of the first skills that an infant learns. This is not easy when you have a huge head relative to your body size. Babies learn a lot about movement by trying to get a view of interesting things, while not keeling over in the process.

Another basic function of trunk alignment is facilitating movements of the arms and legs. Efficient walking, reaching, and squatting all require coordination with the trunk. For example, during a squat, the low back moves into a little flexion, which allows the head to move forward over the base of support. An overhead reach with two hands is facilitated by spinal extension. Reaching with one hand requires side bending or rotation, depending on whether you reach up or forward. Walking involves counter-rotation. Kids usually master the basics of these coordinative patterns at a young age, by which time they have also necessarily developed good fundamentals in postural control.

The postural system also works to protect you from injury. The trunk is home to the spinal cord, many joints, and all the vital organs. If you are about to be involved in a collision, the muscles of the trunk and neck will immediately brace. Even simple tasks like stepping down from a curb require at least some degree of spinal stiffness. If you are not ready for the impact, you can get hurt. But as with many other things, the right amount of bracing is not too much and not too little (and as we will see, far less than commonly claimed).

Good posture minimizes the effect of repetitive mechanical stress. Many common tasks require the eyes to focus in one direction for an extended period, which requires holding the same basic position. To reduce stress, posture is constantly varied in subtle ways to shift the burden from one place to another. This is why we sit in multiple positions, shift weight from one leg to the other as we stand, and generally fidget whenever we are spending more than a few minutes in the same position.

Postural skills are put to a more difficult test in a dynamic context. In gymnastics, surfing, and skateboarding, just staying upright is a major challenge. In sports with an opponent, good posture affords the ability to move in any direction at any moment, which is an overwhelming advantage. This "reversibility" is lost as soon as you are caught off balance, leaning in one direction and committing yourself to only one option.

For the above reasons, optimal posture is not a single anatomical arrangement, but many. Posture needs to constantly change according to current needs for safety, function and comfort. Therefore, the best posture for sitting is not the same as the best posture for standing, or running, or playing golf. There are admittedly some common mechanical elements to each of these postures — verticality and "neutral" spinal alignment are generally quite useful. But there will always be subtle differences based on context.

Further, the best posture for one person is not necessarily the best for another, because everyone has a different structure. In fact, the best posture for you in sitting *at this moment* is likely different from the best posture for you in a couple minutes, because by then you will be a different person, with different levels of muscle fatigue in certain areas, different functional goals, and different levels of accumulated stress in your joints. Fortunately, the postural system is highly sensitive and responsive, so it will know that you need a change, and will cause you to fidget to a slightly different position that is more comfortable and functional.

DYNAMICS OF POSTURE

The trunk is designed for lots of small movement in many different places. The spine has 24 vertebrae that can each move into flexion, extension, rotation, side bending, and sliding. Twelve of the vertebrae attach to ribs, which can articulate independently of the spine. Trunk movements are controlled by a great number of muscles pulling in various directions. Some of them connect vertebrae to their immediate neighbors, while others span nearly the length of the back. Other muscles connect the vertebrae to the ribs, pelvis, head, shoulder blade, arm and femur.

The complexity of this anatomy means that we have virtually infinite options to move or hold the trunk and neck. This is a good reason to be skeptical about common claims that we should always strive to hold the spine in a perfectly straight line. Why would we have so many options for movement if we weren't meant to use them? We are like snakes with arms and legs. Although it's hard to notice when standing still, the trunk's freedom of movement is always in use. For example, as you sit, and shift your pelvis a bit to the right or left, this will tilt or rotate the bottommost vertebrae in the same direction. To keep your head steady, one of the higher vertebrae must compensate by moving in the opposite direction. There are 23 choices of where that can be done. Similar movements of the trunk are occurring every time you reach for a computer mouse, take a breath, or scratch yourself.

Even when postural alignment remains steady, it is never rigid. The head oscillates back and forth over the base of support, constantly making fine-tuned adjustments.[2] Your balance is therefore dynamic, not static. You are always in the process of slightly falling and then recovering. As you tilt a little to the left, muscles on the right side of the body lengthen, and this is detected by proprioceptive sensors in the muscles. These send a signal to the spinal cord, which triggers muscle activity that tilts you back to the middle. The vestibular system also works to keep you balanced. Sensors in the ears detect the slightest movements of the head, and this activates reflexive movements to keep the eyes level and the head balanced.

If your eyes move left in their sockets, this immediately facilitates activity of the muscles that turn your head left. They are helping the eyes find their target. If you put your fingers at the base of your skull, you may be able to feel the muscles respond as you turn your eyes side to side. The spine also tends to follow the eyes up, down and forward. Olympic weightlifters look to the ceiling as they lift, which helps promote movement of the spine into extension. Looking down has the opposite effect. These reflexes are frequently used in yoga, where poses are coordinated with eye movements. While working on a computer, your attention goes to the screen in front of you, and the neck "helps" the eyes by moving the head forward, which tends to slump the chest. If you change your visual attention to be more peripheral, the muscle tone in your neck will reorganize to allow the head to float back over the spine. Scientists have recently discovered that the eardrum of a chimpanzee can move *within the ear* to follow the eyes.[3] The ear is trying to hear what the eyes are looking for. The lesson is that many parts of the body take direction from the eyes. Getting a good view of things is a fundamental task, and the postural muscles self-organize in line with visual constraints. Their activities occur well below awareness in a bottom-up fashion, and are therefore very difficult to control top-down with conscious direction.

Here's a specific example to give you an appreciation for the subtlety of the postural system. The inner ear of a frog (just like a human) detects head tilt. The ear has semi-circular canals, in which there are air bubbles. When the head tilts, the bubbles move, and this triggers tiny sensors in nearby hair cells. The hair cells send a signal to the spinal cord, which needs to know about the head movement so it can activate muscles to remain balanced. So the ear talks to the spinal cord, which is interesting, but even more interesting is that the spinal cord talks back to the ear. Each time the spinal cord executes a forward movement, it also sends a signal to the inner ear, which desensitizes the hair cells, making them less likely to fire. Why? The spinal cord already "knows" the head will be moving, because it just gave the command to walk, so it's telling the ear not to bother talking about it.[4] The point of this story is that there is a lot going on beneath the hood, and we will never know more than the tiniest fraction of it. The system works very well without us trying to control it. According to Nicolai Bernstein, a pioneer in the science of motor control, we should think of the postural system as we would an internal organ. It doesn't benefit from "interference in its business."[5]

POSTURE AND PAIN

Bernstein's advice is very different from what you hear from popular posture gurus and media headlines. They warn we should be paying a lot of attention to posture, constantly policing it to prevent all sorts of problems. If we don't become aware of postural defects and make appropriate corrections, we are likely to develop back pain, "text neck," shallow breathing, and many other ailments. A quick Google search reveals a number of scary headlines from mainstream media sources: "Is Your Posture Killing You?"; "Good Posture: A Matter of Life and Death?"; and "Is Your Smartphone Destroying Your Health?" The answers to these questions are No, No and No.

There are many different schools of thought about how posture should look and what should be done to correct it. One common theme is that slumping is bad, and likely to cause pain in the neck, upper back or shoulders. A slumping pattern is variously called forward head posture, upper cross syndrome, or more recently text neck. Common corrections for these alleged defects include stretching the muscles in the chest, strengthening the muscles between the shoulder blades, and rehearsing a taller posture with various cues like "tuck the chin" or "pinch the shoulders back." These are all versions of the perennial advice to "stand up straight!"

Another concern of postural gurus is alignment of the pelvis and low back. The most common "dysfunction" is too much inward curve (lordosis) in the low back, and/or a pelvis that tips forward in the front. This pattern is called anterior pelvic tilt, lower cross syndrome, or sway back. It is held responsible for back pain, hip pain, tight hamstrings, poor athletic performance, and the unjustified appearance of a beer gut. Common prescriptions to fix this defect include strengthening the abs or glutes, stretching the hip flexors, or spending most of the day bracing the core.

Another popular idea is that postural asymmetry causes pain, because it stresses one side of the body. The symmetry of the pelvis is of particular concern, because it provides the base of support for the spine. Leg length discrepancies are commonly noted, because they will tilt the pelvis. Foot posture is also considered relevant, because this will affect "functional" leg length. Because it's "all connected," some therapists will treat back pain by addressing posture of the foot, or vice versa.

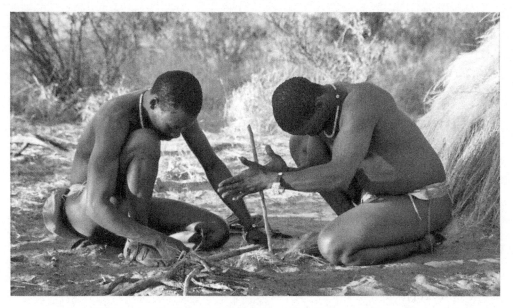

Figure 9.1. Before text neck there was fire-starting neck.

These ideas have intuitive appeal and are advocated by numerous experts. But they are not well supported by evidence and are in many cases flatly contradicted by it. The overwhelming majority of the research on posture and pain does not support a causal relationship. Here are some representative findings from more than thirty years of studies:

- No association between leg length inequality and back pain.[6]
- No difference in lumbar lordosis or leg length inequality in 321 males with either severe, moderate or no back pain.[7]
- No association between neck pain and neck curvature in 107 people over the age of 45.[8]
- No significant difference in lumbar curve, pelvic tilt, leg length discrepancy, and the length of abdominal, hamstring, and iliopsoas muscles in 600 people with and without back pain.[9]
- Teenagers with postural asymmetry, excessive thoracic curve and/or lumbar curve were no more likely to develop back pain in adulthood than peers with "better" posture.[10]

- Pregnant women with larger increases in low back curve during pregnancy were no more likely to develop back pain.[11]
- A review of ten studies found no correlation between thoracic kyphosis and shoulder pain. (But there was less shoulder ROM.)[12]
- Teenagers with slumped forward head postures didn't have more neck pain (although they were more depressed).[13]
- No association between low back pain and spondylolisthesis (a condition where a vertebra has slipped forward, and which is often corrected by fusion surgery).[14]
- In a group of women aged 65-91, those with substantial kyphosis had no more back pain or disability (but they were significantly shorter).[15]
- No association between neck pain and "text neck" as assessed by physical therapists.[16]
- Ergonomic programs do not reduce the risk of a future onset of neck pain, but exercise reduces the risk by half.[17]

Although some studies have found a positive association between measurements of spinal alignment and pain, these are exceptions to the rule, and the correlations are relatively weak.[18] The weight of the evidence is perhaps best represented by a systematic review done in 2008, that analyzed more than 54 studies on the link between pain and posture. Together they did not produce evidence supporting an association between measurements of back to front spinal alignment and pain.[19] Although back pain is associated with scoliosis, this condition refers to relatively large side to side asymmetries that are not present in 98% of the population.[20]

Other relevant studies examine the effects of jobs that involve repetitive use of postures thought to be awkward or stressful. These have found that:

- Sitting at work is not associated with low back pain.[21]

- A systematic review of 35 studies found that occupations that require lifting weights probably do not cause low back pain.[22]

- A systematic review of 99 studies found no good evidence of a causal connection between back pain and occupations that involve awkward postures, lifting, bending and twisting.[23]

- Although occupations that routinely require heavy lifting are associated with increased risk for back pain, the effect size is modest.[24]

The above research indicates that if any correlation exists between posture and pain, it is weak. These results are striking given that many studies have easily found other factors that correlate with low back pain, such as exercise, job satisfaction, educational level, stress, and smoking.[25] Further, even if a correlation between pain and posture does exist, this would not prove a causal relationship. It may be that pain causes bad posture, or that some unknown factor causes both. This is highly plausible. People who are injected with a solution causing back pain will spontaneously adopt different postural strategies to reduce discomfort.[26]

These studies may be surprising, but less so if we remember that people are living things, not machines. Unlike car tires, humans adapt to the stress of uneven alignment. Whatever posture you habitually use is probably one that you have been using for many years, maybe even most of your life. So you have already done a multi-year, everyday workout to get ready for whatever stresses your posture is currently causing. You are trained and ready for the bad posture Olympics.

The second reason that seemingly "bad" postures do not correlate with pain is that everyone has a unique structure, and therefore good posture for one person might be bad for another. As noted in the chapter on structure, the shape and size of the skeleton vary considerably between different people. This fact makes assessing posture according to an objective standard inherently problematic.

Another confusion stems from overrating symmetry as a sign of proper function. Irregularity is to be expected in any biological form. Body parts are not interchangeable legos or Ikea furniture pieces made by factory molds. Wonkiness and asymmetry are part of the plan. If you aren't convinced, play with the phone app that lets you see your face as two symmetrical right halves, or two left halves. For most people, the two faces look distinctly different.

BE A GOOD EXAMPLE

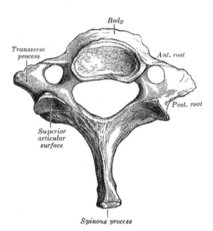

Figure 9.2. A typically asymmetrical vertebra, courtesy of Gray's Anatomy.

While extreme deviations from symmetry are often a sign of a problem, this is not necessarily the case. Do a Google search to see pictures of the very crooked spine of Lamar Gant, an elite powerlifter. If he listened to postural experts about the dangers of loading a bent spine, he would have never managed to break world records in the deadlift.

Based on the above considerations, many international leaders in the treatment of musculoskeletal pain, such as Lorimer Moseley, David Butler, Peter O'Sullivan, and Max Zusman have been asking therapists for years to spend far less time worrying about posture. Unfortunately, the rate of change in practice is very slow.

POSTURE AND CORE STRENGTH

The obsession with alignment of the back is related to another concern — we need core strength to protect it. It is true that core muscles play an important role in preventing unwanted movements. Stability is especially important during activities that create a lot of force on the low back, including heavy lifting, or high-speed bending or rotating.

However, most of life requires only minimal activation of the core musculature. During walking, the abdominals have an average activity of 2-5% of maximal voluntary contraction. Standing requires core muscles to fire at less than one percent. Add more than fifty pounds to the torso and they fire at three percent.[27] During sitting and bending, muscular activation is similarly low. And yet these are exactly the activities that are often very aggravating to people with sensitive backs. Given that these tasks seem to require so little core strength, why is it that they often cause pain, and how will more core strength help?

Although core exercises can reduce low back pain, they seem to work no better than many other treatments, including brisk walking, general exercise, or even exercises directed towards relaxing the core muscles, which is basically the opposite of bracing.[28] It turns out that people with back pain actually use *more* core activation during common movements. They brace their core muscles, so their movements into bending or twisting are "stiffer, slower, less variable and more guarded."[29] Bracing seems to be an instinctive response to pain, an apparent decision by the postural system to limit movements that may be aggravating a tender area. This is probably a good short-term strategy, but it may have costs over the long term.[30] Bracing is energetically inefficient because it requires extra muscle work, and it limits mobility and function in certain contexts. And bracing works by compressing the joints, which may over time be a source of excess stress. Peter O'Sullivan, a physical therapist and back pain researcher, argues that common advice to brace your core during everyday activities may be counterproductive. He often gets clients to feel better by doing less, not more work, with their abs.

Another school of thought says that core strength is not as important as core control. Under this view, subtle errors in timing and coordination of the core muscles may cause instability. The logic is sometimes explained with a car analogy. Most of what keeps us safe while driving is not powerful brakes but using them at the right time. Motor control for the spine became popular after some interesting research by Paul Hodges found that people with chronic low back pain respond differently to postural perturbation, especially in the activation of deep core muscles like the multifidus and transversus abdominus. On the basis of this research, therapists developed highly precise exercises to activate these muscles, including drawing in the navel. Millions of Pilates classes were sold on this idea. However, as with core strengthening, research on motor control for low back pain showed that it works, but not better than other methods. Further, the people who improve on core control programs don't necessarily change the way they move.[31] They feel better, but their mechanics are the same.

PLAYING WITH POSTURE

The research on posture and core strength should not be construed to mean that posture doesn't matter for pain or performance. On the contrary, posture is a fundamental aspect of motor control, one of the first skills that a baby learns. We can barely do anything without a well-organized trunk and neck, and high-level athletic performance necessarily requires high-level postural skills. And when you have pain that is obviously related to maintaining a particular posture, it makes perfect sense to start exploring different ways to organize it. Thus, a better interpretation of the research is that postural organization can't be assessed with simple objective measurements in a static non-functional context. Good posture is complex, individual, dynamic and contextual. It doesn't make sense to measure it with a plumb line, or try to improve it with one-size fits all rules.

A better approach is to explore different postural options and find what works best for you. For example, I have noticed that standing in the same place for long periods of time, as you might do at a cocktail party or museum, will sometimes make my lower back stiff. It feels better almost immediately when I sit for a few minutes. In a slumped position! I have clients that have literally the exact opposite set of preferences, which is why they use a standing desk at work. Fortunately, most of us are attracted to good postural solutions through sensory feedback, and find them without any conscious effort. But this natural learning process can be inhibited by conscious applications of "rules" about which postures are right and wrong. Thus, instructions to brace yourself or stand up straight can be counterproductive, impairing the relaxation, spontaneity and variability that are required for efficient body use. Research shows that fear of movement related to bending or twisting can predict excessive core bracing, reduced postural variability, and bad outcomes in chronic pain.[32] Here's some wise words from the ecologist C.S. Holling: "Placing a system in a straitjacket of constancy can cause fragility to evolve." The problem with common postural advice is that it encourages people to put themselves into straitjackets of constancy, causing them to be more fragile and less resilient.

So what is a better strategy for improving the organization of the systems that control posture? Recall that it is difficult to control complex systems directly in a top-down manner. It's better to think in terms of changing the constraints around which they self-organize. So let's review some potential constraints on posture.

Coordination affects posture, especially during the performance of skilled activities. The trunk needs to help the arms and legs, and without good cooperation, there are postural compensations. Therefore, movements that require good integration of the trunk with the limbs, such as crawling, walking, running and swimming (all locomotive movements) will also tend to improve the organization of the trunk. Postural skill is also about balance, and therefore we might expect it to be improved through activities that challenge balance, like gymnastics, dance or skateboarding. Variability is a key aspect of coordination (we'll discuss this more in chapter ten). Practices like yoga, Pilates, or tai chi develop skills in maintaining a particular alignment under variable conditions. In my previous book *A Guide to Better Movement*, I offer about twenty lessons based on the Feldenkrais Method, which are designed to help you "remember" all sorts of subtle movements in the spine and ribs that you may be neglecting. This can help you explore a broader range of options for staying upright.

Strength and endurance might limit postural options in contexts where fitness is an issue. It is a challenge to hold a safe and functional posture when lifting a heavy weight, running a distance at a brisk pace, or performing a powerful throw. You need strength to resist the forces pulling you out of alignment. But fitness is less likely to affect posture during everyday activities, which require surprisingly little core strength.

Another potential constraint on posture is mobility. For example, you need pretty good range of motion in the hips to sit upright on the ground with the legs extended. If you don't, the hamstrings will pull your pelvis into a backwards tilt, and you will therefore need to round your back to keep your head level. If you improved your hip mobility, your sitting posture would immediately reorganize to make your trunk more vertical, perhaps improving comfort and efficiency. But this change would probably be specific to sitting with extended legs and might not affect other postures.

Posture has a psychosocial dimension. Body language sends social signals about mood and confidence. Teenagers may slouch to look cool. Some people suck in their stomachs to flatten their belly, lift the chest to show dominance, or collapse it to be submissive. On vacation, body language might change to reflect a more relaxed and comfortable mind. I have noticed that my back gets tired after a formal social function where I have to wear a coat and tie. Something about the occasion inhibits my natural movement and literally makes me feel stiff.

Attention and environment regulate posture. As noted previously, one of the reasons you tend to slouch when you look at a computer screen is that it helps you get closer to the object of your attention. If you direct your attention to the wide world around you, to objects both far, near, up, down, left, right and even behind you, your head will naturally move into a more upright position. Next time you are hiking, imagine you are in untamed wilderness, and need to be aware of potential threats coming from 360 degrees. You will notice a spontaneous change in the organization of your trunk and neck.

Pain can be a major constraint on posture. We instinctively move away from positions that hurt us. Many people who have their backs "go out" will find to their surprise they have spontaneously adopted a very crooked posture. The postural system immediately reorganizes to protect a tender area.

What all of this means is that anything you can do to improve your general physical function might also improve your postural organization. Not in the sense of looking more vertical, but in the sense of having a body that is a more functional and comfortable place to live.

10

SKILL

Correct exercise is, in fact, a repetition without repetition.
—NIKOLAI BERNSTEIN

We talkin' 'bout practice.
—ALLEN IVERSON

All day we are solving movement problems, such as finding an efficient and comfortable way to walk, breathe, or reach for a refreshing beverage. We take these skills for granted because we execute them without effort, or even conscious thought. But the information processing required to perform them is staggering. The most sophisticated robots struggle with simple tasks like loading and unloading a dishwasher. To be fair, my eight-year-old is not that good at this yet either.

The Russian physiologist Nicolai Bernstein was one of the first scientists to look at physical coordination as the product of complex systems. He developed his theories in the mid-twentieth century but they continue to be highly influential today, and have inspired a number of other models based in systems theory, including nonlinear pedagogy, dynamic systems theory, and ecological psychology.[1] In this chapter we will discuss motor skill from the perspective of these theories, including the nature of skilled movement, how to improve it through playful and other means, and why movement skill matters for movement health.

COORDINATION AND DEXTERITY

To solve a movement problem, you need to move with coordination, which means the different parts of the body must cooperate in a harmonious way. For example, in a coordinated running stride, all the major joints and muscle groups work together in sync to move you forward. But coordination alone is insufficient for real-world function. A further requirement is adjusting coordinative patterns to fit the particular circumstance, which is always changing. For example, when you run over an uneven surface, you must constantly alter your stride on the fly to avoid tripping or stepping in a hole. Bernstein called this improvisatory skill "dexterity," and recognized it as a higher level skill than mere coordination.[2] A car engine can be coordinated — all its parts can move with a synchronized organization. But it takes a driver for the car to move with dexterity and respond to variable conditions with intelligence. Dexterity is especially important when trying to avoid a predator or catch prey.

How does the body move with dexterity? The traditional answer is that motor control is imposed on the body "top down" by a brain that has all the answers about how to move. These answers are encoded in "motor programs" that specify what needs to be done by every muscle and joint to accomplish a specific task. Bernstein showed this top-down model could not fully account for dexterous movement, which always involves novel elements for which the brain couldn't possibly have any prior programs. Consider the simple act of writing your signature in different ways — one on a check, the other on a blackboard, the other on a blackboard with a towel pinned under your writing arm. The results will be similar, even though the required muscle contractions and joint movements will be completely different, and some will have never been done before.[3] The first signature is done mostly by the wrist and fingers, the second by the shoulder, and the third by the trunk and legs. The only common element is the *intention* to create the result. The intention comes from the higher levels of the brain, but the intelligence that executes this intention is widely distributed all over the body, emerging from interactions between muscles, joints, sensations, reflexes, and feedback from the environment. Through this bottom-up process of self-organization, the final motor pattern will be "soft-assembled" at the moment of execution. Thus, skilled movement involves a kind of "motor wits," or ability to improvise new solutions on the spot. We are more creative than we imagine.

Even in situations where the environmental conditions are exactly the same on each repetition, the need for improvised variability is critical. For example, when expert blacksmiths repeatedly strike a target, they use a slightly different pathway on each swing. Bernstein calls this "repetition without repetition."[4]

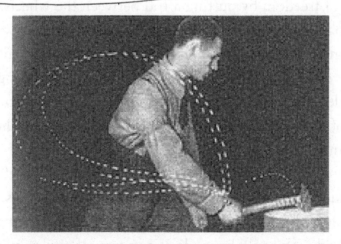

Figure 10.1: An expert blacksmith displays repetition without repetition.

Variations in technique are necessary to compensate for minor path deviations that will inevitably occur as the swing is initiated. These variations require further adjustments, and so on, so that each swing must be subtly different from the previous one. Thus, an essential aspect of hammering skill is the ability to use different coordination patterns to get the same result, and to adjust them on the fly. Novice blacksmiths have less skill in this regard and show less variability in the way they strike the target.[5]

LIKE NOVICE MOVERS

THE DEGREES OF FREEDOM PROBLEM

Although variability in movement is a source of skill and adaptability, it also presents a challenge. The human body has so many different moving parts that getting them all to cooperate is a task of almost unimaginable difficulty. Bernstein called this the degrees of freedom problem.[6]

It is relatively simple to control movement in a mechanical system with only a few degrees of freedom. A door is constrained by hinges, so it can only move back and forth. This makes it very easy to control, provided you can remember whether to push or pull. Driving a car is possible because the four wheels don't move *independently*. We reduce its degrees of freedom by putting a rod between the wheels, constraining them to move in the same direction at the same time.

But human bodies have 360 joints that move independently, and in multiple directions. And there are 640 muscles crossing the joints at odd angles. Imagine the difficulty of controlling a marionette with hundreds of moveable joints and strings. Or think of all the ways you might attempt to dribble a basketball. You could use one or more of the following movements: finger flexion, wrist flexion, elbow extension, shoulder extension, spine flexion, flexion in the hips, knees and ankles. Each of these movements could assist pushing the ball down to the floor. And each could be made at a variety of angles, with different amounts of muscular force, and in combination with other synergistic or opposing movements. Out of all the different options, only a vanishingly small proportion will produce a good result. How does the motor control system find a good solution?

At the outset of learning, novices simplify the degrees of freedom problem by locking certain joints in place.[7] For example, beginning basketball players may dribble by freezing the elbow, and moving mostly from the wrist and shoulder.[8] There are now fewer moving parts, so coordinating their activity is easier. The disadvantage is losing the service of a joint which could help with the task. Freezing a joint is like taking a player off the field to make teamwork easier. Even worse, keeping the benched player frozen requires extra stabilizing muscle work. The result is movement that is energetically inefficient, and robotic in appearance. You can see this style in beginners learning to dance, swing a golf club, or ski. They look stiff and awkward.

When we gain skill, we start to "release" degrees of freedom, letting more joints get involved in the movement. This makes movement appear more smooth, flowing, and graceful.[9] Novice racquetball players start by freezing the wrist, and then gradually releasing it to gain power and versatility.[10] When infants learn how to move, they start in positions where their movement options are highly constrained, such as lying on the floor. They gain more freedom as they sit and crawl, and more still as they stand and walk. During their first attempts at standing, they maintain balance by freezing movement in the knee and ankle, making postural adjustments mostly by movement in the hips. As they develop, they gradually learn to coordinate the whole leg.[11]

From these examples, we can see that movement skill is about being very free to move, but also highly organized at the same time. Great athletes combine stability with flexibility, producing the same basic patterns under a wide variety of conditions. For example, Tiger Woods uses a Tiger-style swing on each stroke. But within the constraints of his signature technique, he is free to alter his swing in a million subtle ways to make necessary adjustments for different slopes, grasses, winds, distances, spins, heights, errors made mid-swing, etc.

Bernstein thought stability could be combined with variation through the use of "synergies" — coordinative patterns of muscle/joint usage that are stable, but which can be combined in different ways to create variety. For example, reaching the right arm forward is almost always accompanied by rotating the trunk left. This synergy can be used as a building block for complex movements like crawling, walking, climbing, throwing, etc. Bernstein's ideas about how different movements are assembled were further spelled out in his theory of four different "levels" of motor control.

LEVELS OF MOTOR CONTROL

Bernstein describes the different levels of motor control as if they were parts of a house that has been in construction for billions of years.[12] The "lower" levels govern basic functions like postural control and locomotion, and the higher levels allow specialized functions like throwing a rock or working with tools. The parts of the nervous system that govern the lower levels are more primitive. They evolved earlier and have less connection to higher level nervous system functions like environmental awareness, conscious attention, and decision making. Lower level skills emerge naturally in infants and young children through play, without any deliberate practice. They are also more fundamental, meaning they are almost always in use, providing a supporting or "background" role for more specialized functions. The higher-level skills are more specific, and only used in certain contexts. To develop them, you need far more conscious attention, practice, coaching and "work." Here is a more detailed (but still very rough) description of the different levels.[13]

Level one: trunk and neck control

The most basic form of motor skill is postural organization. As discussed in the previous chapter, this is one of the first skills an infant begins to master. The neural systems that control it are primitive and started evolving when we were fish in the ocean. As such, they need very little assistance from higher centers of the nervous system. Indeed, work at this level is "almost totally involuntary and largely evades consciousness."[14]

Level two: large multi-joint limb movements

The second level of motor control involves large movements of the arms and legs in coordinated multi-joint patterns. These evolved primarily to serve the purpose of locomotive activities such as walking, running, climbing and swimming.[15] As such, level two movements tend to be cyclical, rhythmic, and repetitive. They are also global, requiring work from nearly every muscle and joint in the body. This is the level where synergies are most important to keep one part of the body constrained to act in coordination with others. For example, when both hips flex, this encourages flexion at many other segments of the body, such as the knees, ankles, and back. The full expression of this global flexion synergy would be going into a fetal ball. The pattern is reversed when both hips extend and you stand tall — extension in one area makes other areas attracted to extension as well. Moving from global flexion to extension is how you get from squatting to standing. Performing the same movement with power creates a jump. Running is basically jumping from one leg to the next. These synergies simplify the process of learning new skills, which are built from combinations of simpler skills.

The attractors for level two movements are wide, meaning they are easy to find, and emerge through self-organization without instruction. In fact, "central pattern generators" in the spine create locomotive movements in mammals and reptiles without any contribution from the brain.[16] This is why humans don't need much coaching in locomotive skills. Arthur Lydiard, one of the most famous running coaches of all time, summarized his thoughts about running technique with the following: "Forget about form."

Although the systems that govern level two movements evolved to serve locomotion, their synergies are used in many other activities that involve whole-body coordination, especially in cyclical movements like cycling, rowing, sawing, or exercises like repeated squats, kettlebell swings, jumping jacks, pushups, pull-ups, rope skipping, etc. Each of these activities is characterized by mobilizing nearly every major muscle group and joint into synchronized patterns of rhythm. This makes them aesthetically pleasing, graceful, even awe-inspiring. Bernstein likens proper coordination at this level to a well-orchestrated symphony.

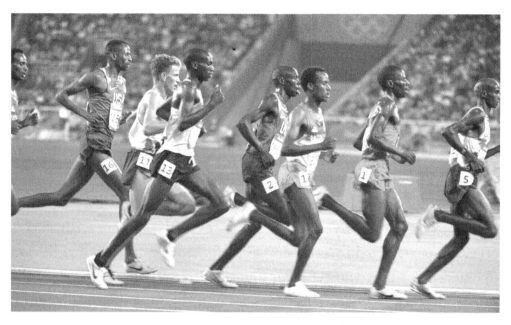

Figure 10.2: A symphony of movement.

Level three: targeted movements

The next level of motor control relates to movements whose purpose is to achieve some specific effect in the environment, such as moving the body (or an object) to a precise location. Unlike the cyclical repetitive movements in the second level, third level movements are usually a singular event, with a clear beginning and end, such as a lift, jump, throw, or catch. They are characterized by crisp, businesslike accuracy and precision, as opposed to the smooth, flowing gracefulness of level two. Throwing a ball to a target is a level three skill.

Level three is an advance from the previous levels in its awareness of the external environment. The lower levels are concerned mostly with movement of one body part relative to the others, while level three perceives the relationship to the outside world. Thus, level three is where merely coordinated actions become truly dexterous.[17] This requires ongoing sensory feedback, especially from the eyes, about whether the movement is achieving its intended purpose. Further, because the processing of visual information depends on conscious attention, mental focus plays a larger role in ensuring proper performance of targeted activities. To hit a baseball (level three), you need to pay close attention to the ball, but running (level two) actually gets less efficient when you focus on the body.[18]

Level four: complex actions *Solve Problems*

Complex actions are sequences of movements that, when linked together, solve a motor problem. If any link in the chain is omitted, the goal is not accomplished. The ability to execute complex actions evolved only recently. It is found only in higher mammals, and even young human children struggle to perform them.

Complex actions are frequently performed by manipulating an object with the hand, which is the most dexterous part of the body. Unlike movements controlled by the first three levels, complex actions are often performed far better on one side than the other. Bernstein uses the example of taking a cigarette and lighter from your pocket, shielding it from the wind and lighting it. This is composed of thirty to forty separate movements, each of which need to be performed properly to achieve nicotine delivery. Most kids under the age of eight would fail in this task, which is probably for the best because they really shouldn't be smoking anyway. When young children attempt more socially appropriate complex activities, such as handwriting, shoe tying, or playing a musical instrument, they quickly fatigue or get bored.

In the context of sport, complex actions are best exemplified by skillful control of a ball or racquet. Elite performance in these areas does not come as "naturally" as movements controlled by the lower levels. Instead, you need to put in thousands of hours of deliberate practice, and probably get some coaching as well. You also need to watch other great players and emulate what they do, because the optimal solutions to the relevant motor problems are not easy to find. You won't just stumble over them with random explorations of the movement landscape, unless you are a prodigy.

Complex actions are highly specific to a certain context — they help you solve one kind of movement problem, but not others. Improving your serve in tennis is not likely to change your performance in any other activities. But an improvement in your running form might help in any sport that involves running. This is one of the reasons complex skills are hard to acquire: the system is not that interested in learning skills that do not have broad application.

How the four levels work together

The four different levels do not work independently — most activities require at least some contribution from each. However, one level will usually play a dominant or "leading" role, while others remain in the "background." For example, running is mostly controlled by levels one and two (postural control and large limb coordination). Level three (targeting) helps to make sure you don't step in a hole or get lost. Classic exercises like the squat, lunge, pull-up, or pushup are similar — most of the challenge is synchronizing the large muscles that work together to produce compound multi-joint movements. Level three makes sure the movements start and finish in the right place — for example achieving a certain depth in the squat. Hitting these targets is usually the appropriate focus of conscious attention. As we will discuss later in this chapter, directing attention inward will tend to disrupt the organization of levels one and two.

In activities such as putting a golf ball, or shooting a gun, the higher levels are very active, while the lower levels basically just make sure you hold a stable posture. Shooting two guns while flying through the air and doing the splits to avoid bullets involves lots of work from all four levels, which is why we like to watch this type of thing in slow motion. It is possible to be quite skilled at one level, and relatively less so at another. This is why we might see a talented musician with poor posture, or an amazing runner who can't catch a ball. It's why Shaquille O'Neal was a hall of fame basketball player who couldn't beat a guy off the street in a free throw contest. Now that we've discussed the nature of movement skill, we will turn our attention to how we acquire it through play and work.

THE GAME IS THE TEACHER

One simple takeaway from a systems-based approach to learning movement skill is that the "game is the teacher." This means we learn by *doing*, not consciously applying advice from an expert about how to move. The right environment for learning is a playfield not a classroom. In fact, we don't have much conscious knowledge of how to move at all. When you lift a wineglass, do you know how much you need to activate the biceps versus the deltoid? As you take a step, what is the proper timing for the activity of the peroneus longus? Even biomechanists have only a vague idea, and they are no better at wineglass lifting and walking than anyone else.

Imagine you are driving on the highway and want to switch lanes to the right. How *exactly* do you turn the wheel to do that? Think for a minute before reading on! Most people answer that you turn the wheel to the right and then back to neutral. But this action would actually send you on a rightward diagonal that would soon take you into the guardrail. The solution is to turn the wheel to the right, then back to neutral, *then to the left*, and then back to neutral. Next time you're in the car, watch what your hands do to confirm. (Watch the road too.)

Even less intuitive is turning a bicycle to the right. What do you do with the handle bars? A turn to the right is initiated by turning the handle bars slightly *to the left*. This allows you to *lean* the bike to the right, which is actually what gets you changing direction to the right. Would kids learn to bike faster if they were told that opposite-side-leaning is the trick to controlling a bike? This information would probably just be confusing. In most cases, the best teacher is the activity itself.

Another famous example demonstrating the complexity of a seemingly simple task is the "outfielder problem." It asks: how does a baseball player solve the problem of catching a fly ball hit some distance from where he is standing? Our first assumption might be something like this: when the ball is hit, the outfielder estimates the speed and trajectory of the ball, makes a prediction about where the ball will land, and then runs directly to that spot in a straight line as fast as possible, making adjustments along the way. This is not how it's done. A simpler and more effective method is to get your eyes on the ball, and then run so that the ball stays in your visual field and continually looks as if it is moving the same speed.[19] Players don't need instruction to find this technique. In fact, dogs use it to catch frisbees.[20] So how would a baseball coach teach someone to shag fly balls? About 95% of the job is arranging for the student to catch fly balls, at a moderately challenging level, using variable heights and speeds, and occasionally reminding the student to keep their eye on the ball.

Thus, good coaching is about providing the athlete with "problems not solutions." The game is the teacher. If you set up the right constraints — the right game, in the right environment, with the right motivation, with the right opponents and teammates — the systems that control movement will self-organize, and you will learn the right skills. The job of a coach is to help arrange these optimal learning conditions.

EXPLORING MOVEMENT LANDSCAPES

Another simple analogy for motor learning is exploration of a "landscape" in search of solutions. Here's a quote from developmental psychologist Esther Thelen about how babies learn to move:

> The course of learning for each baby appeared to be one of **arousal, exploration, and the selection of solutions from that exploration space.** In basic form, the developmental pattern

is this: The presentation of an enticing toy is arousing and elicits all sorts of nonproductive actions, and very different individual actions in different babies. These actions are first, quite literally, all over the place with no clear coherence in form or direction. But by acting, **by movements that explore the whole range of the movement space,** each baby in his or her own unique fashion, sooner or later makes contact with the toy— banging into or brushing against it or swiping it. **These moments of contact select some movements in this space, carving out patterns that are then repeated with increasing frequency.** Over weeks, the cycle repeats—arousal by the sight of some toy, action, and occasional contact.[21]

So babies learn by semi-random exploration, and then repetition of what works, until effective movements become habits. As stated in Chapter 3, movement habits can be represented as attractor wells on a landscape.[22] The attractor wells for fundamental movements like reaching, crawling, and walking are very wide. With any amount of exploration, babies find them easily.

You can appreciate the attractiveness of a basic movement pattern like contralateral walking by trying to do it the "wrong" way. Try walking homolaterally — with the right arm moving forward as the right leg steps. It feels unnatural but is possible with conscious effort. But as you speed up, the contralateral pattern becomes almost obligatory. The architecture of the muscles, bones and connective tissues, combined with primitive nervous system reflexes, make contralateral walking a movement pattern that is not only easy to find but hard to avoid.

Other movement solutions, especially complex actions built from sequences of sub movements, are not so obvious at all, and can only be found with thousands of hours of search, and probably a qualified guide as well. Playing the piano or performing a double backflip are not things that people tend to figure out all on their own after some playful experimentation. They require imitation of other experts, breaking down the sequence into smaller parts, and proper coaching.

FUNCTIONAL AND NON-FUNCTIONAL VARIABILITY

Although variability is a source of dexterity, not all variations in movement are good. Roger Federer hits his forehand a bit differently on each stroke, but the variations are not random. You will never see him hit the ball lefty, or with the side of the racket. Instead, Federer displays "functional variability," which means the differences in each stroke contribute to good outcomes, as opposed to just being errors.[23] Part of his learning process was finding out which aspects of his forehand technique needed to be the same on each repetition, and which need to be modified.[24]

Frans Bosch calls the stable aspects of a good technique "attractors," and the variable aspects "fluctuators." When attractors are highly functional, they establish what are often called good "fundamentals." A fundamental is a component of a movement technique that is present in every successful repetition, whether by the same player in different conditions, or by different players in the same condition. For example, Bosch argues that the fundamental position of the shoulder for throwing is ninety degrees of abduction. Although you will see athletes throw in many different ways (e.g., different trunk angle, stride length, wind up, follow through, objects) they will almost always hold the arm straight out from the trunk during the most powerful parts of the movement.

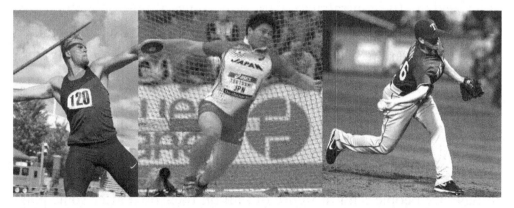

Figure 10.3 Different trunk angles but same arm position relative to trunk. Some other common elements: a sequence of stepping toward the target, trunk rotation, arm action, wrist action and follow-through.

This fundamental throwing position is easy to learn because it is highly attractive. Any time you move the arm with lots of force, you will gravitate to the abducted position, because it is the safest and most powerful position for the shoulder. In other words, throwing with good form is relatively "natural" for humans. Hitting a baseball or tennis ball is less natural, therefore discovering good fundamentals is not as easy. The stable aspect of a swing should be the movement of the hands and shoulders along a certain trajectory. The variation should come from changes in the position of the lower body and trunk — this is what puts you into position to hit the ball.[25] Novices tend to use the reverse strategy, keeping the lower body stationary, and moving the hands to get to the ball. This means they lose the powerful connection to the trunk, and wave at the ball ineffectively. Over time they will learn, by repeating swings under variable conditions, which parts of the swing should remain stable, and which need to be varied.[26]

Coaches influenced by systems thinking often incorporate variability into practice to speed the learning process. For example, runners benefit from training at different distances, speeds, inclines, surfaces, with and against resistance. Powerlifters use different foot positions, kinds of resistance, speeds, surfaces, stances, ranges of motion. Soccer can be played with variable field size, number of players, and rules. In each case, the basic strategy is to practice moves that are "the same but different" or to engage in "repetition without repetition." The players slowly learn what is essential and what is optional. This makes technique robust, applicable in many contexts. Variable practice may be especially valuable for novices, who need to do more exploring to find good techniques.[27] For example, one study shows that novices learn faster if they make more mistakes, which are "grist for the learning mill."[28]

To summarize this complicated information, let's return to a simple rule: the game is the teacher. To make sure your learning is multi-dimensional and comprehensive, remember to occasionally change the rules of the game. You don't want to change the rules so much you are playing a completely different sport, but enough so you are challenging your abilities in slightly different ways, encouraging new adaptations, and finding robust solutions.

PERCEPTION AND ACTION

You need information to solve movement problems. When a gymnast attempts a backflip on the balance beam, she needs accurate perception about her body position relative to the beam. Perceptive skill is required to perform even simple tasks like walking. If we misperceive the location of the foot relative to the ground (perhaps by failing to see a hole or ridge in the sidewalk), the leg muscles will not activate at the right time to absorb the impact, which may cause a fall. So if we want to move well, we need to perceive well.

The reverse is also true, and this is a bit more confusing. We also need to move well to perceive well. This insight comes from James Gibson, who noted that perception is a very active process. Think of an eye moving left and right to see its surroundings, or hands pawing around in the dark to find a lost object. These are "epistemic" movements — their purpose is to gather information that will help you solve some problem.[29] You are moving to perceive.

All movements serve at least some epistemic purpose. Each time we reach out with our foot to take a step, we are searching for sensory feedback from the ground that will tell us about the surface we are walking on, and the exact position of the foot relative to the ankle, knee and hip. When golfers are getting ready to hit a ball, they waggle their club in some idiosyncratic manner. They aren't rehearsing the swing, but trying to get a feel for the relationship of the hands, shoulders, hips and club. When pool players draw back their cues to strike the ball, they are searching for a position that gives them a good sense of the cue in the hand. Good technique in side shuffling in basketball or tennis keeps the head level, so the eyes can accurately track the opponent or ball. As discussed earlier, outfielders accurately perceive ball

flight through accurate body movement.[30] The right movements deliver
the right information at the right time.   *FALLACY of REDUCTIONISM*

Here's a reason this matters. Because perception and action work
together, you can't effectively practice a movement skill unless you
simultaneously practice the related perceptual skills. For example, you
wouldn't train to catch fly balls by practicing running one day, and
then stationary visual ball tracking the next. But similar mistakes occur
in athletic training. A good example is the use of agility drills, where
the athlete runs around cones in rehearsed patterns. In sport, agility is
about changing running direction *in response to some visual cue,* such
as the movement of an opponent, or the ball. When you run around
cones in choreographed patterns, the perceptual challenge is removed.
The resulting practice might be effective in developing a specific kind
of fitness in the lower body, but it will not build links between perception and action that are critical for real-life agility. When a running
back is trying to evade tacklers, he must constantly monitor the environment and make decisions about where to go. More importantly, he
must maintain the balance and "reversibility" to change directions if
the need arises. When you know exactly what movements you need
to perform in advance, you aren't challenged to improve anticipation,
dexterity and balance.

Based on these considerations, coaches influenced by systems thinking try to make sure practice sessions keep perception and action "coupled." In other words, practice should look more like a game, and less
like a repetitive drill. For example, in soccer, small-sided games (e.g.,
four on four), are preferred to choreographed passing drills. For evasive
agility, the most fundamental training is some version of the most basic
game of all, played by every animal and child — tag.

These ideas can be applied to make common exercise programs
more engaging and functional. Running on a treadmill at exactly the
same speed, mile after mile, is a very different experience from running
on a trail, where you must scan the surroundings, and make adjustments
to speed, posture, and foot placement. The trail is an environmental

constraint that changes the way you self-organize — it causes you to spontaneously adopt a technique that will make you more dexterous. Your physical activity now involves a component of skill and visual attention, making it a richer and more multidimensional experience.

Similarly, resistance training with free weights or bodyweight is a different experience from applying force to machines that move along predetermined pathways. The machine removes all perceptual demands related to sensing the position of the weight, and making corrections to ensure balance is maintained. This is why people are rarely passionate about machine training, but often develop a keen interest in power-lifting, kettlebells, gymnastics, bodyweight training, Pilates, yoga, or other kinds of exercise that involve a perceptive challenge. When action stays coupled with perception, movement feels more playful, interesting, and meaningful.

THE ROLE OF ATTENTION

Perception is affected by attention, which acts like a spotlight on sensory informaiton. If you're at a crowded cocktail party, your ears receive auditory information from many different conversations, but you can only "hear" one at a time: the one to which you direct your attention. Each time you shift your attention, a different conversation becomes understandable, but others get tuned out.

There are many "conversations" going on in your body all the time. As you sit here reading this book, mechanoreceptors are continually reporting mostly irrelevant sensory information to the brain: that your shirt is touching your back; that your ribs are moving with each breath; that there is pressure against your seat; that your hamstrings are in a lengthened position. Most of this sensory information does not turn into a conscious perception, because your attention is directed elsewhere. But as soon as you attend to a certain body area, you feel what's happening there, because attention acts like a spotlight on sensory information.

Attention also affects motor performance. Obviously, if you don't pay attention to the ball, you have less chance of hitting it. What about attending to certain key movements of the body? For example, trainers often tell athletes to "fire your glutes," or "hinge at your hips," or "keep your back straight," or "lift your knees." What is the effect of these attentional cues on performance?

Gabriel Wulf is a leading authority on the effect of attention on performance and learning. She studies the difference between two basic types of focus: internal and external. Internal attention is directed at the body, such as the wrist action during a throw, or the extension of the hips during a jump. External attention is directed outside the body, such as a target for throwing, or an overhead object to reach for during a jump. Wulf's research shows that in a wide variety of circumstances, external attention is superior for performance and learning.[31]

For example, one study found that unskilled sprinters ran faster when they focused on pushing their feet into the ground, compared to extending the leg behind them.[32] External cues have also been found to improve performance in jumping, agility, and strength.[33] They are associated with increased movement efficiency and running economy, and reduced heart rate, muscle activation, and perceived exertion.[34] For example, runners feel like they aren't working as hard when they focus on distance, as opposed to gait mechanics. External cues have also been shown to improve dart throwing,[35] golf shot accuracy,[36] balance, and posture.[37] In each task, it seems better to focus on the end result of the task, and not the specific body mechanics used to achieve it.

These results are striking given the seeming similarity between the attentional cues. In one study, Wulf asked subjects to perform a balancing task on a machine that simulated skiing.[38] The internal group was instructed to "exert force on the outer foot" while the external focus group was told to "exert force on the outer wheels" of the machine. The cues sound pretty much the same, but the external group had better performance. Why? Wulf argues that internal focus "interfere[s] with automatic motor control processes that would 'normally' regulate the movement." By contrast, external attention allows the body to "naturally self-organize, unconstrained by the interference caused by conscious control attempts."[39] In other words, trying to control your movement top-down interferes with bottom-up processes that are far more intelligent.

Folk wisdom agrees. When a pro basketball player is shooting the lights out, the announcer might say he is "unconscious." I can recall that as a young tennis player, my excuse for losing was often that my opponent played "out of his mind." In the movie Caddyshack, Chevy Chase said the key to golf is to "be the ball." The opposite mindset is getting too much in your head. Research confirms that internal attention is associated with choking, even in experts.[40] Excessive self-consciousness tends to cause paralysis by analysis and freezing of degrees of freedom. Nick Winkleman has pointed out that an expert choking moves like a novice learning. You may have experienced this yourself — an activity that feels natural and effortless in practice suddenly feels stiff and awkward under pressure. It has been speculated that learning a skill with an internal focus makes it more likely to revert to this attentional strategy under pressure, increasing the chances for choking.[41]

Thus, the role of the conscious mind during performance should be maintaining mental and emotional focus on the end goal, not thinking about the movements to achieve them. This sounds like the flow state described by Csikszentmihalyi, which involves the feeling that actions are happening effortlessly. When the pressure is on, getting into a flow state is not easy, but the pathways for access are built during non-stressful play.

Here's an important caveat: this doesn't mean we should never have internal attention during performance or practice. Internal attention may be occasionally useful with novices, and in learning complex movements with many different parts. You can be sure that most pro golfers are well aware of exactly what their body is doing at many points during a swing. But during performance, and a good deal of their most useful practice, they focus on goals not methods.

MOVEMENT "DYSFUNCTION" AND THE COMPLEXITY OF "CORRECTION"

We are now going to shift gears away from performance and towards pain. What is the role of dexterity in preventing injury? There is no doubt that moving with poor body control at high speed or under heavy load can cause traumatic injuries like muscle strains or torn ACLs. When large forces are involved, you need good mechanics to handle them safely. What about less intense activities like running? Are you at greater risk of repetitive stress injury if your gait pattern is less than ideal? For everyday movements, do you need to have "correct" form in squatting, bending, reaching and breathing? Could "dysfunction" in these basic movements cause pain in the knee, back or shoulder?

Most physical therapists would answer yes. The most common models for pain treatment are aimed at curing "kinesiopathology," which literally means "disease caused by movement." Here's a quote from Shirley Sahrmann, one of the most influential physical therapists of the last few decades:

> Maintaining or restoring precise movement of specific segments is the key to preventing or correcting musculoskeletal pain . . . **When movement deviates from the ideal, it is reasonable to assume that degenerative changes will likely occur. An analogy is found in the wheel movement of an automobile.** For optimal rotation, wheels must be aligned and in balance.[42]

Note the machine analogy! According to Sahrmann, persistent pain is frequently caused by movement "impairments," which can be identified with objective assessments, and fixed with motor education. For example, back pain may be blamed on poor form in bending, and treatment would involve exercises that help train optimal technique.

Similar ideas can be found in "corrective exercise," which is concerned with using proper technique in basic exercises like squats and lunges. The assumption is that fixing "dysfunctions" in basic move-ments will reduce the chance of injury and increase performance *even outside the gym.* One of the most popular proponents of corrective exer-cise, the physical therapist and CrossFit coach Kelly Starrett, explains that his philosophy is based on the simple premise that everyone should be able to perform basic "maintenance" on themselves. Note again the promise to find and fix mechanical problems.

These advocates for correcting movement have a good point. It is indeed true that movement habits determine which body parts receive mechanical stress. Some ways of moving are obviously safer and more efficient than others, and we should strive to move as safely and effi-ciently as possible. So the basic premises of the corrective model are sound. But in practice, corrective methods often ignore the complexity and variability of movement, and the body's ability to adapt to stress over time.[43] This is revealed in a substantial body of research that is simi-lar to the research on posture discussed in the previous chapter. It shows:

1. Movement patterns that are commonly alleged to be dysfunc-tional are not correlated with pain or increased injury risk;

2. Treatments aimed at correcting specific dysfunctions often work no better than general exercise; and

3. Corrective methods may create good results even when no "cor-rection" occurs.

In other words, the benefits of coordination training for pain are probably more about playing with movement than fixing dysfunc-tions.[44] Here is a brief review of some highlights.

Low back pain

Low back pain is often treated by trying to improve coordination of the hips and trunk. For example, under Sahrmann's Movement Systems Impairment model, a therapist might assess a patient's coordination in forward bending. If there is not enough flexion in the hips, and too much flexion in the low back, this might be diagnosed as a "lumbar flexion impairment." The opposite problem is "lumbar extension impairment," where limited movement into hip extension is compensated by extending more in the low back. Treatments seek to correct any impairments that may be contributing to pain. It sounds like a reasonable approach, and it can help with pain. But several studies have found that it works no better than general strengthening and stretching exercises around the area of pain, without any effort to correct specifically diagnosed problems in coordination.[45] In other words, you can treat a flexion impairment in the exact same way as an extension impairment and get the same result. Other studies have made similar findings about other motor control approaches to back pain treatment.[46] This has led many experts to conclude that movement patterns often labeled as dysfunctional are probably healthy and normal variations.

Another common treatment for pain involves correction of "muscle imbalances." For example, pain in the hips or low back is often blamed on weak glutes and overactive hamstrings. Glute strengthening is a very popular treatment, and nearly all my back pain clients have been told to try it. But the biomechanical rationale is weak — research shows that pain is often correlated with *more* glute activity not less.[47] Thus, strengthening the glutes may help with pain, but the mechanism is probably not correction of an "imbalance."

Pilates and yoga have been touted as good treatments for low back pain, partly on the basis of their ability to improve coordination in the hips and core. But research into these exercises for treatment of low back pain shows the same basic pattern: they help for pain, but no better than general exercise.[48]

Knee pain

Knee pain is frequently blamed on dysfunctional movement patterns, such as inward collapse of the knee, or outward tracking of the patella. The relevant biomechanics are complex, but it has been established that knee pain is associated with weakness in the quads and hips.[49]

Exercises to strengthen these muscles are effective for knee pain,[50] but the benefits probably don't depend on changing biomechanics at the knee.[51] For example, simple knee extensions on a machine, which are often derided as being "non-functional," help with knee pain.[52] The mechanism is probably changing tissue health, load bearing capacity, and/or perception.[53] Or perhaps exercise helps painful areas reactivate a stalled recovery process, or escape a loop of persistent pain sensitivity. Based on this view, physical therapists such as Greg Lehman recommend that people spend less time worrying about subtle biomechanical flaws, and more time working to improve the general health and function of the relevant joint. This relatively simple strategy is sometimes referred to as "just load it."

Shoulder movement and pain

Therapists often assess the movement of the scapula while the arms are raised overhead. "Winging" of the scapula is considered a potential cause for shoulder pain (and unsightly as well). But several studies have shown no correlation between ugly scapular movement and pain.[54] Others find that motor control treatment for shoulder pain is effective, but the benefits do not correlate with actual changes in shoulder movement. In other words, the people who felt better after treatment did not on average move any better (and some even appeared to move worse!)[55]

A recent study argues that most scapular movement patterns alleged to be dysfunctional probably represent "normal movement variability."[56] Because shoulder movement is so complex, it is unlikely that we can divide its movements into right and wrong with simple objective tests. Acknowledging the complexity of the shoulder can actually make treatment simpler. Instead of trying to ensure that movement conforms to one ideal stereotype, therapists should simply work on improving the shoulder's general mobility, strength and functionality, and let the system self-organize. Greg Lehman refers to this approach as developing comprehensive capacity.

Running Corrections

Runners are often told to shorten their stride, increase their stride rate, and avoid heel striking in favor of a mid-foot or forefoot strike. This advice is featured in the popular POSE and Chi Running methods, and the best seller *Born to Run*. Kelly Starrett offers a particularly strong opinion on this issue: "If you're heel striking when you run, you have to stop. It's eating you alive."[57] Is heel striking as bad as flesh-eating bacteria?! The research creates no cause for alarm.

Heel-striking is not associated with increased injury rate,[58] and is the most energy efficient way for most people to run.[59] This is why the vast majority of runners, including close to 75% of *elite* half-marathon runners, are heel-strikers.[60] Further, trying to correct running form is unlikely to prevent injury, and will often cause runners to be slower and less efficient.[61] Several studies have asked runners to change their habitual stride length, and found they required more oxygen to run at the same pace.[62] For example, sixteen triathletes were given expert supervision in the POSE method, which recommends a transition from heel to forefoot strike. At the end of twelve weeks, forefoot striking was still less efficient.[63] In fact, simply directing attention to running form, without effort to change it, is associated with reduced efficiency.[64]

Advocates of barefoot running claim that heel striking is only more efficient in cushioned shoes. It is true that minimalist footwear tends to encourage a mid or forefoot strike, but this does not result in less injury or better performance. Although a forefoot strike will usually reduce mechanical stress to the knee, it also increases stress and injury to the foot, ankle and Achilles.[65] The lesson is that there are many different ways to run, and they all have different costs and benefits. You have the best chance of finding what works best for you if you play with as many as possible, by running on different terrains, at different speeds, in different footwear, etc.

Pronation is another controversial issue. It has long been argued that *excessive* pronation of the foot is bad, and may contribute to overuse injuries at the foot, knee, hip and even back. However, after decades of study, it appears that overpronation *might* be a *weak* risk factor for medial tibial stress syndrome and knee pain.[66] Even if overpronation was meaningfully correlated with injury risk, this would leave open the question of whether gait correction would reduce it. If the tendency to pronate is caused by the bony structure of the foot and ankle, this is not something that can be changed. Perhaps pronation can be altered by orthotics? It is true that orthotics can reduce injury risk. But it doesn't seem to matter whether the orthotic is custom-made or bought off the counter.[67]

You could also try to purchase a shoe that is specifically designed to reduce pronation. However, research indicates that shoes don't always have the biomechanical effects intended by the designers. For example, cushioned shoes do not reduce ground impact force, because the body seems to "want" a certain amount of feedback from the ground, and it will work harder to get it through a cushion.[68] According to Benno Nigg, a leading expert on the connection between running shoes, gait, and injury, this is because the foot has a "preferred movement path."[69] Thus, when runners wear different shoes, they usually continue to follow the path they prefer.[70] Following this logic, the best shoes to prevent injury are those that facilitate the preferred pathway, and this can be determined by simply picking the shoe that is most comfortable. In one of Nigg's studies, runners who were allowed to pick their shoe inserts based on comfort experienced less injury than the control group.[71] Based on this study and more than four decades of looking at the complexities of the issue, Nigg's practical advice is simple — try on four to five pairs of shoes, jog around the store, and pick whatever shoe feels best.

General movement skills and the Functional Movement Screen

The Functional Movement Screen (FMS) was developed by the physical therapist Gray Cook to help athletes prevent injury and improve

performance. It includes seven assessments of basic movement patterns
— three directed at the lower body (squat, lunge, single leg balance);
two for core stability (pushup and anti-rotation); and one for shoulder
mobility. Each movement is scored on a scale of 0-3 according to simple
objective criteria. Movements scoring below two are considered dysfunctional and should be corrected with specific exercises before being
loaded in any significant way. One of Cook's basic principles is that one
should not "put fitness on dysfunction" because this increases the risk
of injury. This idea is not supported by the weight of the evidence. Low
FMS scores are not correlated with injury risk,[72] and have little or no
ability to predict athletic performance in a variety of ways, including
agility, vertical leap, sprint times, and elite athletic status.[73] This is probably because FMS skills do not transfer to the field of play.[74] In other
words, the FMS does not test dexterity, but a specific form of rehearsed
coordination.

PLAYING WITH MOVEMENT SKILL: OPTIONS NOT CORRECTIONS

So does all this research mean that dexterity doesn't matter for preventing injury or treating pain? I think a better interpretation is that
dexterity is probably important, but very hard to measure with a few
objective tests, and not easily "fixed" with simple recipes. Bernstein
likened coordinated movement to the harmonious playing of a symphony. Could we assess the quality of Mozart with a few measurements? Probably not. We can easily distinguish Beethoven from Bieber
through aesthetic intuition, but such judgments would not be precise
or universal. Something similar is probably true about good movement.
We know it when we see it, but we don't know (yet!) how to measure it.

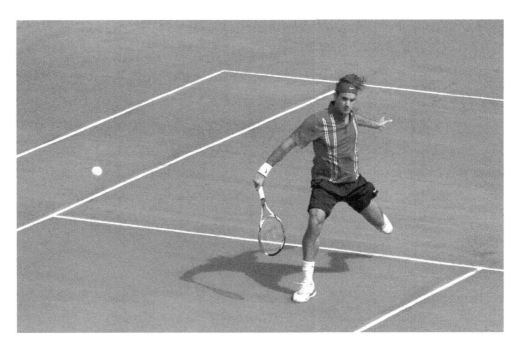

Figure 10.4: We don't need formal assessments to know that Federer moves well.

Another problem with the corrective model is its potential to demonize movements that are normal, healthy and useful, like heel striking or flexing the lower back in a forward bend.[75] We will discuss the dangers of kinesophobia (fear of movement) and nocebos (the opposite of placebo) in the chapter on pain.

Despite these weaknesses, it would be wrong to conclude that corrective methods have nothing useful to offer. Although recommendations about how to move the "right" way are usually not mandatory, they may point the way towards unexplored options. For example, squatting with the spine in a perfect neutral position is not necessary (or even possible), but it's an interesting challenge that may improve body awareness and functional variability in squatting. Running on your forefoot is not something you *must* do, but it's a reasonable thing to try if you are having problems with your current technique. Similarly, there is no reason to fear bending at the low back when you go to pick up a sock. But if bending hurts, you should be curious about whether improved hip flexibility might help. If that doesn't work, move on to something else. If you have shoulder pain with reaching, exercises to improve control of the scapula are a logical treatment option. But it is only one choice among many. Thus, we can look to corrective exercise for ideas on how to play with movement skill, **remembering that the** **goal should be to expand our repertoire of movement solutions, not reduce them.** We should think in terms of options not corrections.

11

PAIN

PSALM 139: 14

We are wonderfully and fearfully made.
—LORIMER MOSELEY

Pain is an opinion.
—V.S. RAMACHANDRAN

Pain is a conscious experience created by complex patterns of activity in the brain. The brain has more than 100 billion neurons, and each are connected by synapses to an average of 7,000 neighbors. When one neuron fires, this either inhibits or excites immediate neighbors, which changes the behavior of other neurons, and so on. This extreme connectivity means that neurons can fire in a near infinite number of combinations, estimated to be greater than the number of atoms in the universe.

The patterns of brain activity going on in your head right now help determine how you move, think, and feel. Some create the feeling of seeing blue sky, others a sky that is slightly darker. Some will cause you to experience the taste of chocolate. Others trigger memories of the past, or fears about the future. And some patterns of brain activity create the feeling of having pain. This activity is widely distributed across many different brain areas, including those related to memory, expectation, fear, goals, and movement. Thus, there is no single "pain center" in the brain, and no simple switch that can be thrown to stop it.

Most pains arise in the following manner: A body part is damaged, the damage is detected by sensory receptors near the site of the injury, and a danger signal is sent to the brain. The brain reads the signal, perceives the need for a protective response, and reacts in a way that creates pain. Therefore, we can think of pain as the output of a highly sophisticated alarm system.

GOOD FLOW CHART

Despite the complexity of the physiological events that lead to pain, not all pains present a mystery. Pain in your foot is easily explained if you find a splinter right where it hurts. You know why your knee hurts today if you fell on it yesterday. Even when the cause for pain is not obvious, it might be discovered through a detailed medical examination, or an x-ray, which might find a broken bone or torn ligament. Thus, not all pains are complex, and a reductionist "biomedical" treatment approach works very well in many cases, especially those involving a specific pathology.

But the origin of some pains is more elusive. Think of all the times you have been unable to explain why some particular pain comes or goes. You wake with a crick in your neck, or suddenly have your back go out. Knee pain suddenly starts to hamper your running, even though you are running the same route you've done easily for years. You get intense pain between the shoulder blades at work, which stays around for a few weeks, and then fades away for no reason. You have aching in the hip that moves around - down to the butt and back of the leg, or up to the sacroiliac joint. Or you have widespread pain in multiple areas that changes intensity and location every hour, every day. The ambiguity of these examples is typical of a significant percentage of chronic pain complaints, including the majority that come to my office. In fact, I have personally experienced most of the above problems for at least a few weeks. In my twenties, I had persistent back pain, and now at age 50 I have been free of this problem for a couple decades. It's not about getting older. On average, back pain becomes more prevalent until age 60 and then declines.[1] What this all means is that pain often cannot be blamed on local tisue damage. Instead, it may be caused by something more complex — an interplay between a variety of factors, many of which relate to the pain alarm system itself.

As we'll see in this chapter, the pain system is adaptive, always changing its level of sensitivity to potential threat. Sensitivity can rise or fall dramatically over short periods of time, even as the physical tissues remain in substantially the same condition. Unfortunately, these facts are often ignored in mainstream medical practice, which tends to focus on structural reasons for pain. Thus, when patients have pain that cannot be traced to a specific injury, they are often given implausible explanations, such as poor posture, bad alignment, a weak core, getting old, tight muscles, "scar tissue," or dysfunctional movement patterns. In previous chapters, we reviewed the evidence calling these diagnoses into question. In this chapter, we will look for some alternatives that recognize pain's potential complexity.

Here's a quick caveat before we get started. **Even if pain cannot always be explained by specific local pathologies, you should always have an expert look for them. Make sure to consult with a qualified medical provider before applying any of the advice in this book to treat pain.**

THE FUNCTION OF PAIN

[handwritten margin note: AN ATTEMP TO PROTECT OURSSELF IN THE PRESSNCE OF A PERCEIVED THREAT]

The purpose of pain is protection: if you sprain your ankle while running, pain gets you to stop running and start limping, so the ankle can rest and heal. Like the stress response described in chapter four, pain is about helping the body respond to a perceived emergency. Indeed, some experts view pain as one component of the stress response.[2]

The protective function of pain is clarified by imagining life *without* pain. Some people are born with congenital analgesia, meaning they can't feel any pain at all. At first glance this sounds like a good problem to have, but the costs far outweigh the benefits. People with congenital analgesia bite through their tongues while eating, get third degree burns without noticing, and don't realize their leg is broken until it collapses under their weight.[3] They don't fidget when they sit or stand, because they never feel uncomfortable. As a result, their joints accumulate repetitive stress, and they eventually develop severe degenerative joint disease at young ages. Tragically, they often die young.

These facts make clear that pain is fundamental to health, function and survival. A useful analogy is that pain is part of an internal alarm system that detects physical threats and initiates protective behaviors. Here's a revealing question: What level of sensitivity would you set the alarm for someone who you really cared about? If you set the alarm to a hair trigger, they will receive strong protection against physical dangers, which is good. But they will also get false alarms, and experience more pain, which is bad. If you reduce the sensitivity of the alarm, they won't be bothered with trivial threats, but they run a greater risk of failing to prevent a catastrophe. So as with any other physiological condition in the body, there are trade-offs in setting the sensitivity of the pain alarm system. It is constantly modulating its behavior to balance these considerations, based on its reading of many different factors.

Huh!

BASIC PAIN PHYSIOLOGY

Following is a brief discussion of basic pain physiology, focused on how the system changes its sensitivity to threatening stimuli. We will start by looking at three different levels[4] of the nervous system: (1) the peripheral nerves, where potential threats are detected; (2) the spinal cord, where sensory information related to threat can either be amplified or suppressed; and (3) the brain, where the meaning of the sensory information is interpreted in light of other evidence, and decisions are made about whether pain is necessary for protection. After looking at how these different parts of the nervous system work in isolation, we will look at how they communicate, and then expand our view further to the nervous system's interaction with other protective systems like the endocrine system and immune system. The details are somewhat complicated, but when put together they form a big picture view of pain that is fairly simple and common sense.

Peripheral Nerves: Threat Detection

Sensory receptors called nociceptors are located at nerve endings all over the body. They detect potential threats, and can be triggered by mechanical force, temperature change, and chemical conditions related to inflammation, injury, or excess muscle work. When the nociceptors are triggered, they send a signal that may or may not reach the brain, prompting it to consider whether pain is necessary to protect the area.[5]

Nociceptors have a firing threshold — a light touch to your arm will *UNLESS ALLODYNIA* not activate them, but a firm smack will. The threshold can be lowered by several mechanisms, especially the presence of inflammation. This will cause "hyperalgesia" — when something hurts more than it should. You probably know from personal experience that even a soft touch to an inflamed area like a sunburned shoulder or sprained ankle can cause serious pain. When the inflammation subsides, the sensitivity of the injured area should return to normal. However, nociceptors may be able to retain "memories" of past injuries. During periods of heightened sensitivity, they can undergo changes that make them more reactive to similar trauma in the future.[6] This means that the second time you sprain your ankle, you might get the same damage, but even more nociception and pain.

Nociceptive signals can also arise from the middle of a nerve trunk, as opposed to its ending. This is called ectopic nociception, because it arises in the "wrong place."[7] This confuses the higher levels of the nervous system, because they don't know where the signal originated. Therefore, if a nerve is irritated near its root, you might feel it closer to the nerve's ending. This is one of many reasons why knowing where it hurts doesn't necessarily tell you where the problem is.

The dorsal horn: Screening threat signals

Nociceptive signals travel toward the spine, where they meet the dorsal horn of the spinal cord. The dorsal horn acts as a "gate" that can suppress or amplify danger signals. I think of it as a middle manager collecting information from low level employees, deciding which issues to ignore, which to solve immediately, and which to report to the boss.[8] For example, when you sit on a hard surface, nociceptors will report a potential problem with your rear end, but you probably won't feel any pain because the dorsal horn will either ignore it, or take care of the problem by getting you to fidget in your seat, transferring the pressure of sitting to some other area.[9]

The sensitivity of the dorsal horn can be increased, making it more likely to report danger signals to the brain. This is called central sensitization, and it may play a key role in many cases of chronic pain.[10] Central sensitization may also cause pain to spread, because the dorsal horn receives signals from other peripheral nerves in the area, so their danger signals are amplified as well.

SECONDARY HYPER- ALGESIA

Central sensitization is a normal and healthy response to injury.[11] When the dorsal horn learns of a problem, it turns up the volume on any related bad news. As the injury heals and nociception levels reduce, the dorsal horn should return to a baseline level of sensitivity.[12] However, like the peripheral nerves, it may be able to learn from experience, retaining "memories" of past trauma, and an enhanced sensitivity to similar stimuli.[13]

Descending modulation

Descending modulation occurs when the brain acts to change the sensitivity of the dorsal horn, thereby either suppressing or amplifying nociception.[14] Recall the metaphor of the middle manager — descending modulation is the boss letting the manager know which issues are important. Lorimer Moseley states that descending modulation is a way for the brain to "second-guess" the periphery about the threat posed by a particular stimulus. It makes sense for the brain to second-guess because it has more information about what is actually a threat and what is not. This advantage may come from memories, general knowledge, or other sensory input. Imagine feeling a slight tweak in your back during a heavy deadlift, and then remembering you had a similar feeling last year right before having two weeks of back pain. On the next set, your brain will probably be listening carefully for potential danger signals. That's called descending facilitation.

The opposite process is descending inhibition, where the brain is not interested and doesn't want to hear it. The brain knows that many activities which create significant nociception are actually healthy, such as vigorous exercise, getting a deep tissue massage, or sprinting from a dangerous predator. In each case, the brain wants to encourage the activity that is creating the nociception, and therefore blocks the danger signals. This is accomplished by what pain educator David Butler calls the "the drug cabinet in the brain" — cannabinoid and opioid substances that descend the spinal cord and block the upward flow of nociception. These drugs are powerful enough to provide full pain relief from catastrophic injuries, which many people won't feel at all during an emergency. Triathletes are known to have especially powerful pain inhibitory systems.[15] This allows them to somehow endure and even enjoy events that normal people would consider the worst form of punishment. They have excellent internal drug cabinets. In various chronic pain conditions, the descending inhibition system doesn't work very well. Thus, people with fibromyalgia, irritable bowel syndrome, or TMJ typically don't respond well to vigorous exercise, or deep tissue massage, and it will very often make them feel worse.[16] This unfortunate circumstance makes playing with movement much more challenging, because finding the goldilocks window between too much and too little physical stress becomes extremely small.

PAIN AND THE BRAIN

When nociceptive signals reach the brain, the pathways of neural activation become far more variable and complex. Many brain areas activate in parallel, including parts that are involved in sensory discrimination, emotion, fear, memory, cognition, and movement. These are collectively called the pain matrix or the neuromatrix.[17] When they behave in a certain way, we feel pain. This is in some ways a mystery — no one really knows how and why neural activity in the brain turns into a conscious experience.[18] But we have a good idea about the *purpose* of the neural activity associated with pain. According to Lorimer Moseley, the brain is processing information related to threat, essentially asking "how dangerous is this really?" and deciding whether pain is necessary for protection.[19] To do that, it considers all available evidence related to threat, as well the environmental, social and functional context. This is why so many different parts of the brain are involved in creating pain. It also explains why so many factors affect pain perception aside from nociception, including other sensations, emotions, cognitions, and expectations. Here's a brief review of some of the research detailing the impact of these factors on pain.

Sensory information

The eyes are a good source of information about threat to the body, and seeing is believing. When you watch a horror movie, your body reacts, even though you aren't the one getting stabbed. There is an interesting documented case of a construction worker visiting the emergency room in terrific foot pain after a nail went through his work boot. After removing the boot, it was confirmed that the nail had actually gone between his toes.[20] The connection between pain and visual input has been confirmed in controlled studies as well. For example, a red rod applied to the skin feels more painfully hot than a blue one of the same temperature.[21] Needle injections hurt more if you look at the needle compared to the arm.[22] Forward bending is less painful when you do

it while looking in a mirror.[23] And visual illusions about the appearance of a joint have been shown to modulate pain in a wide variety of
conditions.[24]

The sense of touch (mechanoreception) also has significant effects
on pain, and usually serves to reduce it. This is why so many different
touch therapies are effective short-term pain treatments, including massage, ultrasound, kinesiotape, foam rolling, or just good old-fashioned
rubbing an owie. The mechanism is basically distraction – non-threat-
ening sensory input gets the attention of the nervous system, especially
if it is novel or interesting, and this diverts attention from nociception,
making it more likely to be ignored.[25]

Emotion

Pain has both an emotional and sensory dimension. The emotional
aspect is the "badness" of pain that causes suffering and motivates
us to avoid it. The sensory aspect is the feeling that this badness has
a certain location and intensity. We know these variables are distinct
because some people experience one without the other. Pain asymbolia
is a condition where pain doesn't feel bad.[26] When people with this
condition sustain an injury, they accurately sense it, and will describe
the associated feeling as "pain." But the pain is not unpleasant, and
they are not motivated to avoid it. In other words, they have pain that
doesn't hurt. How can that be? The answer seems to involve damage to
certain parts of the brain associated with emotion.

Even if you don't have the kind of brain damage that lets you feel
pain that doesn't hurt, you may be able to dissociate pain from suffering to some degree. Have you ever noticed that some pains are
more unpleasant than others, even though they have similar intensity?
Personally, I find that even a mild pain in the neck will drive me crazy,
while serious pain in my foot doesn't really bother me that much. This
distinction between the emotional and sensory dimensions of pain
might explain why some people actually enjoy certain kinds of pain,

or why Buddhists say that pain is inevitable, but suffering is optional. In fact, many people with chronic pain live quite well. They will tell you that their pain does not cause them a great deal of distress, and certainly does not stop them from doing what they want to do.

Based on the foregoing, it should not be surprising that pain is affected by emotional state. Chronic pain is correlated with persistent negative mood, and depression seems to predict the development of chronic pain.[27] Further, when people are induced to have negative moods in the lab, chronic low back pain increases, and pain tolerance to a new stimulus decreases.[28]

Cognition and expectation

The way you think about your pain can change it. If you believe it is caused by a dangerous condition, such as cancer, it may hurt worse than if you believe it is part of a natural healing process.[29] Expectation has a particularly strong effect. As any magician knows, we perceive in accordance with our expectations, and this is true for pain as well.[30] The classic example is placebo, which is nothing more than the pain-killing effect of expecting benefit from an inert treatment. One of the physiological mechanisms that causes the placebo effect is descending inhibition of nociception, discussed in the previous section. Another is reduction of anxiety, which tends to increase pain.[31] Placebo's evil twin is nocebo, which occurs when expecting pain acts as a self-fulfilling prophecy. Catastrophizing (which means expecting worst-case outcomes) is a risk factor for transitioning from acute to chronic pain.[32] But optimism and self-efficacy — the beliefs that your pain can improve and that you are the one who can improve it — are predictors of recovery.[33]

Therapeutic pain education is aimed at changing false beliefs that may be contributing to pain or preventing recovery.[34] For example, you won't feel very optimistic about recovering from pain if you think it is caused by irreversible joint degeneration. Nor do you want to get moving if you think exercise will cause more "wear and tear" on the joint. For some people, getting rid of these unhelpful beliefs through education is an important part of recovery.[35]

Here's an important caveat related to the role of the brain in pain. None of this means that pain is in your head, that pain is not real, that pain is your fault, or that you can simply think pain away with the right mindset. The processes in the brain that create pain are largely unconscious and therefore hard to control. We can hope to affect them through attention, education, mindfulness, and other cognitive behavioral methods. But we should never think that pain is someone's fault.

A SYSTEMIC VIEW

We have so far discussed pain physiology mostly in terms of how the nervous system processes information related to threat. Several other systems help protect the body. The endocrine system is central to the stress response, and the immune system is needed to heal injuries. Richard Chapman has argued these systems work so closely with the nervous system in protecting the body that they should be viewed as one "supersystem," whose function is to coordinate defensive responses to injury, including the creation of pain. When the supersystem is functioning well, it behaves according to a basic pattern, which is highly useful under a wide variety of circumstances:

1. An injury occurs, and threat is detected;
2. The protective systems become more active and sensitive, leading to higher levels of inflammation, pain sensitivity, and/or stress hormones;
3. The injury heals, and the threat is countered;
4. An "all clear" signal is issued;
5. The protective systems return to a baseline level of vigilance.

To execute this pattern, each subsystem performs specialized activities, and these are coordinated through a chemical "language" spoken by peptides, hormones, neurotransmitters, cytokines, endocannabinoids, and other messengers. As noted in chapter four, one of the hubs for communication between the major defensive systems is the HPA axis (hypothalamus, pituitary gland, adrenal gland). Feedback between the different systems keeps their activities balanced and adaptive. For example, the nervous system won't respond well to an injury without the right signaling from the immune system, and vice versa. This connectivity means that if one system becomes dysregulated, others will change their behavior in response. This is why chronic health problems often travel together, and frequently involve pain.

For example, you are at increased risk of chronic pain if you have autoimmune disease, irritable bowel syndrome, depression, anxiety, PTSD, and insomnia.[36] Notably, women are more likely than men to suffer from *all* these conditions. Back pain is associated with sleep disturbance, stress sensitivity, and mental health.[37] Pain in one area is associated with pain in other areas, indicating a systemic cause.[38] Thus, people with multiple pain sites are at increased risk of developing back pain.[39] Fibromyalgia[40] describes a cluster of symptoms that often run together, such as: pain in multiple areas; numbness and tingling; fatigue; cognitive impairment; and high sensitivity to various forms of mild stress.[41] The cause is unknown, but researchers suspect some form of dysfunction or imbalance in one or more of the immune system, nervous system, autonomic system, or the HPA axis.[42] Fibromyalgia is associated with depression, anxiety, PTSD, and autoimmune disease.[43] Once again, it affects more women than men.

Almost every one of the above conditions involves a heightened state of defensive behavior. Recall the "surviving" versus "thriving" dichotomy discussed in chapter four. The body is always choosing whether to defend against short-term threats, or to make "optimistic" long-term investments in the future. Pain, anxiety, depression and stress-sensitivity may be specific manifestations of a general pattern of defensiveness and hyper-vigilance.[44] There are few specific treatments for these conditions that work significantly better than general health interventions like exercise, sleep, and stress reduction. For example, aerobic exercise is an effective treatment for depression, and may work as well as drugs or therapy.[45] For chronic low back pain, the most effective treatments are exercise, cognitive behavioral therapy, and education about pain.[46] Similar conclusions have been reached about chronic musculoskeletal pain in general.[47] Thus, the best evidence for treating persistent pain points towards improving general health, as opposed to fixing specific "issues in the tissues." Recovery is about executing the relatively simple (but not necessarily easy) strategy discussed in chapters four and five — expose yourself to a healthy level of physical stress, reduce mental and emotional stress, and maximize recovery time. In short, do everything you can to let your body know it's strong, safe, resilient, and capable.

CENTRAL AND PERIPHERAL CONTRIBUTORS TO PAIN

This chapter has focused on pains that are complex, but some pains are relatively simple, caused primarily by local tissue damage. This is most obviously true in the case of acute injury. When injuries occur, the protective systems become active, they take care of the problem, and then things return to normal. When pain persists for longer than it should take for the injury to fully heal, this increases the chance that pain is no longer about "issues in the tissues," but persistent elevated sensitivity in the nervous system, especially higher levels like the dorsal horn or the brain. In other words, the cause for the pain may now be more central and less peripheral.[48]

How can you tell the difference? Just because you can't find a peripheral cause for pain doesn't mean it doesn't exist. Further, peripheral and central causes for pain can co-exist, one feeding the other. Therefore, persistent pain may be hard to explain, and diagnoses should only be made by qualified medical professionals. However, there are some general patterns that may be informative. Pain is more likely to involve a significant central component when the following factors are present:

- There is no specific pathology that explains the location of pain.
- Pain is not well-located and moves around.[49]
- Pain is poorly correlated with mechanical stress on the painful area.[50]
- Pain is correlated with emotional stress, mood, sleep, fatigue, or other symptoms.[51]
- There are multiple painful sites throughout the body.[52]
- There are other complex chronic health conditions such as depression, anxiety, chronic fatigue, fibromyalgia, migraine, IBS, TMJ, autoimmune disease, endocrine disorder, or medically unexplained symptoms.[53]

By contrast, if pain is focused in one area where there is known tissue pathology, the pain varies with mechanical stress in that area, and is not correlated with other symptoms, the pain may be driven primarily by peripheral issues. But even here, there may be an element of complexity! For example, Achilles tendinopathy is a good example of a local problem that may have central components. It originates with damage to the tendon caused by overuse combined with inadequate recovery. Pain is usually well-located right in the area of tissue damage, and the pain gets worse when the area is stressed. The most effective treatment for Achilles tendinopathy (and many other tendon conditions) is resistance exercise that stresses the tendon *at an appropriate level*, so that it can adapt and get better at withstanding load.[54] However, it is still unknown whether the treatment works by changing the structure of the tendon, the nervous system's sensitivity to load in the tendon, or both.[55] **Fortunately, we don't always need to know the specific mechanism to get a good result.** It is often sufficient to remember the basic principles of stress and adaptation discussed in chapter four: the body adapts favorably to stress in the right kind and amount. Thus, a relatively simple strategy of "just load it" is often an effective way to treat pain in a local area when pain is related to movement.[56] If you challenge a tendon to do what it was meant to do at the right level[57] of intensity, it will tend to get healthier, more functional, and perhaps less painful as well. The function of a tendon is relatively simple — handling tensional loads. Therefore, any exercise that applies a tensional load to a tendon is a potential treatment option.

The function of the shoulder is a bit more complex — it needs to be strong, mobile, coordinated, and stable. This gives us a good idea about the best way to treat shoulder pain — try to make it stronger, more mobile, coordinated, and stable, without aggravating the pain.[58] This is a reasonable treatment approach for shoulder pain, and many other kinds of "local" musculoskeletal pains. Greg Lehman calls this developing comprehensive capacity. If you have pain in the hip, knee, foot, or back, try improving the ability of these structures to do what they were meant to do — move through functional ranges of motion with coordination, and handle the associated loads. If it hurts to load the joints at one angle or movement pattern, find another that is less challenging. For example, hamstrings might be painful to load at full stretch, but can work very hard without discomfort in mid-range or shortened positions. Shoulders might hurt during abduction but easily handle flexion. Developing functional ability in one position is a step in the direction of improving the full range of motion. I think of it as slowly retaking territory that has been lost. Go as far as you can, establish a base of support at the frontier, and then try to go further next time. If you can't retake the territory from one angle of approach, try another. Even if this strategy doesn't help with pain, at least you end up with a better functioning hip, knee, foot, or back.

STRESS + RECOVER = HEALTH
(LOAD)

In conditions where the problem seems more systemic, and less about a specific body part, what needs to be "loaded" (or perhaps unloaded) is the movement system as a whole. As discussed in chapter five, healthy physical activity tends to beneficially organize every major system in the body, because they are all involved in one way or another in helping us move. You can also improve general health by getting adequate amounts of sleep, eating a healthy diet, avoiding excessive drug use or smoking, minimizing emotional stress, working to develop a positive attitude, and engaging in meaningful activities at home, work, and with friends. None of these interventions are likely to "fix" a specific problem in the body, but they are all capable of helping the body evolve into a healthier state.

SIMPLE MODELS FOR COMPLEX PAIN

The philosopher Alfred North Whitehead said: "The only simplicity to be trusted is the simplicity on the far side of complexity." Following are a few models for pain that I hope Alfred would find trustworthy.

The neuromatrix model is shown in figure 11.1.[59]

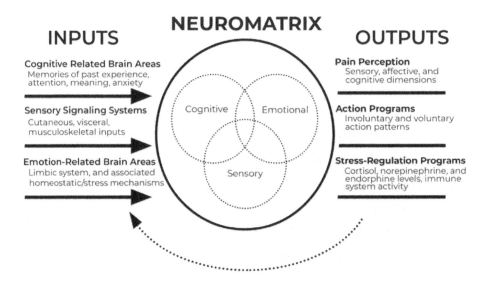

Figure 11.1: The neuromatrix model of pain, adapted from Ronald Melzack.

The "neuromatrix" is in the middle, and is simply the network of brain areas involved in creating pain. The "inputs" to the network are sources of information relevant to physical threat. They are divided into thoughts, emotions or sensory signals. The meaning of the inputs is interpreted by the neuromatrix. If it perceives threat and the need for a protective response, it creates one or more of the "outputs" on the right side of the diagram. These include feelings like pain, movements such as bracing or limping, or stress responses like altered immune or endocrine system activity. The outputs immediately become new inputs into the system, and the process repeats in slightly altered form.

I think this model is useful because it highlights several important points: pain is multi-factorial; it depends on perception; the brain is a key hub for information processing; and pain is part of a larger pattern of self-protection that also includes changes in the immune system, endocrine system and musculoskeletal system. The model also helps identify some possible ways to modify pain, to wit: **the inputs on the left of the diagram (thoughts, emotions and movements) are potentially under our control.**

We can focus on these inputs more directly by looking at other models for pain that are oriented towards patient education and treatment. For example, we can visualize all of the different variables that might be making pain better or worse with some version[60] of the bucket model, discussed in chapter 4.

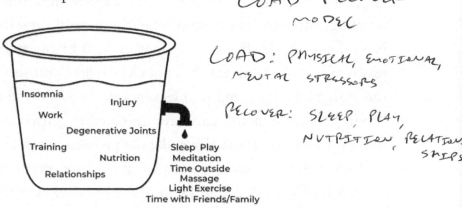

(handwritten annotations) LOAD - RECOVER MODEL

LOAD: PHYSICAL, EMOTIONAL, MENTAL STRESSORS

RECOVER: SLEEP, PLAY, NUTRITION, RELATIONSHIPS

Figure 11.2. A simple way to think about pain, when pain is complex.

This image can help you identify potential treatment strategies when there isn't any *one* obvious target to aim at. Or you could think in terms of the movement health model presented in chapter one. The different dimensions of movement health — structure, fitness, mobility, posture, skill, social and physical environment — are constraints around which the body and its defensive systems self-organize. Some of these constraints are generally overrated for pain, others are underrated. But each provides some opportunity to play with different variables that may affect pain.

COMPLEX PROBLEMS, WICKED PROBLEMS, AND PAIN HABITS

Complex problems, including those related to pain, are not necessarily hard problems to solve. Recall the classic example of a complex problem discussed in chapter four — raising a toddler. Toddlers are self-organizing, and therefore gravitate toward healthy behaviors as long as you provide them with good common-sense parenting. Complex pains are similar, often resolving on their own after a few weeks of common-sense self-care.

However, some complex problems are *extremely* difficult to resolve. Systems thinkers call these "wicked problems." Examples include poverty, political gridlock, the opioid crisis, a broken health care system, or a failing marriage. The system is behaving badly, and the bad behavior is reinforced by feedback loops that make it highly stable. Because the problem is multi-factorial, it is not clear where you should intervene in the system. Further, many interventions, especially those directed at "fixing" a single factor, can have unintended consequences, activating feedback loops that actually make the problem worse.

Unfortunately, some persistent pains are properly classified as wicked problems. We said before that physical activity tends to help with pain. What if physical activity makes pain worse? Sleep and a positive attitude are also helpful, but what if the pain is making them impossible? There are certainly no easy answers to these questions.

The challenge of persistent pain has been noted by many experts. Herta Flor, a neuroscientist, compares persistent pain to a memory that is hard to forget.[61] The physical therapist Louis Gifford uses a similar analogy, likening it to an unpleasant advertising jingle that gets stuck in your head. Vania Apkarian, a professor of physiology at Northwestern University, considers chronic pain to be in the nature of a habit that is hard to break.[62] These metaphors explain certain aspects of persistent pain quite well, and also suggests what solutions might look like. As discussed in chapter three, the "habits" of a complex adaptive system can be visualized with an attractor landscape. Figure 11.3(a-d) illustrates how pain sensitivity levels might change with injury.

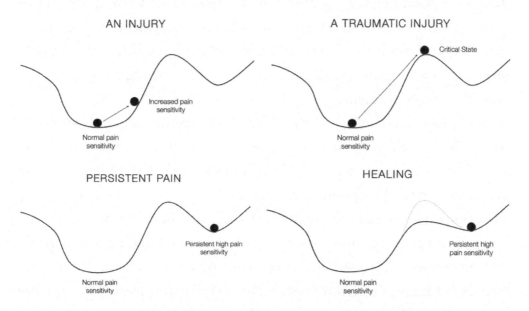

Figure 11.3 (a) a healthy response to injury; (b) a traumatic injury causes a critical state; (c) a phase shift to persistent pain; (d) a chance to break the pain "habit."

Before an injury, the ball is in the well corresponding to a normal level of pain sensitivity. (See Figure 11.3a). When an injury occurs, inflammation and other aspects of the protective response push the ball up the hill to a position representing an elevated level of sensitivity. But this position is temporary, because the injury should heal, and the ball will be attracted back down to the bottom of the well.

Now let's imagine a more traumatic event, such as a car crash, divorce, or major illness. This is a shock to the system, and the ball is knocked all the way up to the top of the hill in figure 11.3b. The system is now in a critical state: the ball may roll left, back to its initial state; or maybe it will roll right into a new attractor well, representing an elevated level of sensitivity, shown in figure 11.3c. This would be a phase shift in the system — a new normal is established. How do you shift back? Perhaps the new attractor well is not deep, so the new normal is not stable. Random noise in the system will eventually perturb the ball back to the healthier attractor well. The healing stimulus might be anything — a good massage, a weekend vacation, some yoga, a trip to the gym, or lots of walking. The efficacy of these treatments is less about specifics, and more about just perturbing the system in some way, getting it to reset to a more adaptive state. It's like turning a computer on and off to fix a problem.

But what if continued efforts to reset the system fail, and pain persists? That would suggest the new attractor well is relatively deep, or that pain has become a habit. This presents a greater challenge — old habits die hard. The good news is that habits can in fact die. Drug addictions may persist for many decades, but they can be overcome. Long-standing political conflicts can be resolved. Trauma can heal, and people who have suffered from chronic pain for many years can recover.[63] I know this from personal experience and from talking with many others. Wicked problems can be solved. But they are not fixed with a single intervention. Positive change is slower, more organic, a process of evolution. Every day our experience transforms us into a slightly different person with a different set of attractors and habits. (See Figure 11.3d). Over time, hyper-vigilant protective systems can slowly shift back to a more relaxed set point, especially when they are supported with rest, stress management, positive mindset, and healthy forms of challenge. It's hard to rush biology, so this doesn't happen overnight. But people heal and change all the time.

Perhaps science will someday find a simple fix for wicked pain. Until then, make sure to keep playing with movement.

RESOURCES

Visit BetterMovement.org for resources and readings lists on each of the subjects in this book, including play, stress, complexity, fitness, strength, endurance, perception, skill, and more.

PICTURE AND ILLUSTRATION CREDITS

Figure 1.1, Image by Carolyn Silvernail.

Figure 3.2, Public domain via Wikipedia Commons.

Figure 4.1, Image by Carolyn Silvernail.

Figure 6.1(a), Skateboarder picture by Ricky Aponte, Creative Commons license.

Figure 6.1(b), Parkour picture by Marco Gomes, Creative Commons license.

Figure 7.1, Picture of hip bones by Joe Dully, courtesy of Paul Grilley at paulgrilley.com.

Figure 7.2, Scoliosis picture from Library of Congress, public domain.

Figure 7.3, MRI chart by Todd Hargrove, adapted from Brinjiki (2015).

Figure 7.4, Public domain, via Wikipedia Commons.

Figure 8.1, Picture of cheetah running by Gregory Wilson, Creative Commons license.

Figure 8.2, Picture of hunter-gatherers squatting by Aino Touminen, public domain.

Figure 8.3, Picture of hip bones by Joe Dully, courtesy of Paul Grilley at paulgrilley.com.

Figure 9.1, Picture of vertebrae from Gray's Anatomy, public domain.

Figure 10.1, Picture of blacksmith in public domain via Wikipedia Commons.

Figure 10.2, Picture of runners by Tim Hipps, Creative Commons license.

Figure 10.3(a), Javelin thrower picture by Koji Kawano, Creative Commons license.

Figure 10.3(b), Picture of discus thrower by Pierre-Yves Beaudouin/ Wikimedia Commons/CC BY-SA 4.0.

Figure 10.3(c), Picture of baseball pitcher by Keith Allison, Creative Commons license.

Figure 10.4, Picture of Federer by Lihian Zhang, Creative Commons license.

Figure 11.1, Image by Carolyn Silvernail, adapted from Ronald Melzack.

Figure 11.2, Image by Carol Silvernail.

Figure 11.3(a-d), Diagram by Todd Hargrove.

ABOUT THE AUTHOR

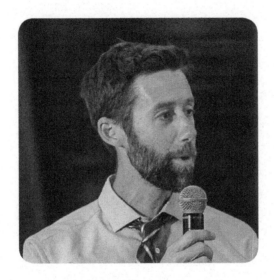

Todd Hargrove is a former attorney, author, blogger, speaker, massage therapist and Feldenkrais Practitioner.

His first book is called *A Guide to Better Movement: The Science and Practice of Moving With More Skill and Less Pain.*

You can follow him on Facebook (Better Movement), Twitter (@ toddhargrove) and his blog at BetterMovement.org

He lives in Seattle with his wife and two daughters.

ENDNOTES

INTRODUCTION

1. Piercy et al. (2018). The Physical Activity Guidelines for Americans. JAMA, 320(19), 2020.

2. Lee et al. (2012). Effect of Physical Inactivity on Major Non-Communicable Diseases Worldwide: An Analysis of Burden of Disease and Life Expectancy. The Lancet 380(9838), 219–229.

3. Hoy et al. (2014). The Global Burden of Low Back Pain: Estimates from The Global Burden of Disease 2010 Study. Annals of the Rheumatic Diseases. Jun; 73(6), 968-74.

4. Moore et al. (2017). Metabolic Syndrome Prevalence by Race/Ethnicity and Sex in the United States, National Health and Nutrition Examination Survey, 1988-2012. Preventing Chronic Disease, 14, E24.

5. Gray (2011). The Decline of Play and The Rise of Psychopathology in Children and Adolescents. American Journal of Play, 3(4), 443–463.

6. Jayanthi et al. (2013). Sports Specialization in Young Athletes: Evidence-Based Recommendations. Sports Health, 5(3), 251–257.

7. O'Sullivan et al. (2016). Unraveling the Complexity of Low Back Pain. Journal of Orthopaedic Sports and Physical Therapy 2016; 46(11), 932-937.

8. See the following for examples: Foster et al. (2018). Prevention and Treatment of Low Back Pain: Evidence, Challenges, and Promising Directions. The Lancet, 391 (10137), 2368–2383; O'Sullivan (2016); Smith et al. (2014). An Update of Stabilisation Exercises for Low Back Pain: A Systematic Review with Meta-Analysis. BMC Musculoskeletal Disorders, 15(1); Ferreira et al. (2007). Comparison of General Exercise, Motor Control Exercise and Spinal Manipulative Therapy for Chronic Low Back Pain: A Randomized Trial. Pain, 131(1–2), 31–37.

9. This is called the Dunning Krueger effect. I wrote a blog post about this subject here: https://www.bettermovement.org/blog/2017/experts-versus-gurus-whats-the-difference

10. Glouberman et al. (2002). Complicated and Complex Systems: What Would Successful Reform of Medicare Look Like? Commission on Future of Health Care in Canada, Paper No. 8, (July), 1–37.

11. Maher et al. (2017). Non-Specific Low Back Pain. The Lancet 2017, 389: 736–47; O'Sullivan (2012). It's Time for Change with the Management of Non-Specific Chronic Low Back Pain. British Journal of Sports Medicine, 46(4), 224 LP-227.

12. Recovery is associated with optimism and self-efficacy, and negatively correlated with catastrophizing. See e.g., Marcuzzi et al. (2018). From Acute to Persistent Low Back Pain: A Longitudinal Investigation of Somatosensory Changes Using Quantitative Sensory Testing — An Exploratory Study. Pain Reports, 3, 1–10; O'Sullivan (2012); O'Sullivan (2016). Further, a "just load it" approach to treating pain is frequently effective. See chapters ten and eleven.

CHAPTER ONE: MOVEMENT HEALTH

1. Huber et al. (2011). How Should We Define Health? BMJ 343, d4163–d4163.

2. With these ideas in mind, groups like the World Health Organization usually describe health in reference to multiple factors, such as: relative freedom from disease; physical, mental and social well-being; resilience and adaptability to various forms of stress; the ability to independently perform meaningful functions like acquiring skills, maintaining relationships, doing a job, and otherwise fulfilling personal potential. See Huber et al. (2016). Towards A 'Patient-Centered' Operationalisation of the New Dynamic Concept of Health: A Mixed Methods Study. BMJ Open 6, e010091.

3. Lindström et al. (2005). Salutogenesis. Journal of Epidemiology and Community Health, 59(6), 440 LP-442.

4. Engel (1977). The Need for A New Medical Model: A Challenge for Biomedicine. Science (New York, N.Y.), 196 (4286), 129–136.

5. Kiely (2017). Periodization Theory: Confronting an Inconvenient Truth. Sports Medicine, 48, 753.

CHAPTER TWO: PLAY

1. Graham et al. (2010). Current Perspectives on the Biological Study of Play: Signs of Progress. The Quarterly Review of Biology. Vol. 85.

2. Graham (2010).

3. Carrera-Bastos et al. (2011). The Western Diet and Lifestyle and Diseases of Civilization. Research Reports in Clinical Cardiology, 15; Lloyd et al. (2011). Evolutionary Mismatch and What to Do About It: A Basic Tutorial. 2011 Sep 25. Available from: https://evolution-institute.org/wpcontent/uploads/2015/08/Mismatch-Sept-24-2011.pdf.

4. Dennis (1970). Play in Dewey's Theory of Education. Young Children 25 (4), 230-35.

5. Gray (2011). The Evolutionary Biology of Education: How Our Hunter-Gatherer Educative Instincts Could Form the Basis for Education Today. Evolution, Education and Outreach, March 2011, 4 (1), 28–40.

6. See the Wikipedia entry on "Minimally Invasive Education." https://en.wikipedia.org/wiki/Minimally_invasive_education#The_experiment

7. There is research showing that athletes who spend more time in "deliberate play" versus "deliberate training" are considered more creative on the field. Wormhoudt et al. (2017). The Athletic Skills Model: Optimizing Talent Development Through Movement Education. 1st Edition. Routledge.

8. Uehara et al. (2018). The Role of Informal, Unstructured Practice in Developing Football Expertise: The Case of Brazilian Pelada. Journal of Expertise 2018. Vol. 1(3).

9. Llenas (2017). Vitilla, Dominican Stickball Using Broomstick and Bottle Cap, Starts Hitting in U.S. Fox News. https://www.foxnews.com/sports/vitilla-dominican-stickball-using-broomstick-and-bottle-cap-starts-hitting-in-u-s

10. "For most sports, early diversification is more likely to lead to success . . . intense training in a single sport to the exclusion of others should be delayed until late adolescence to optimize success while minimizing injury, psychological stress, and burnout." Jayanthi et al. (2013). Sports Specialization in Young Athletes: Evidence-Based Recommendations. Sports Health, 5(3), 251-7.

11. For examples, see Graham (2010); Bateson (2013) Play, Playfulness, Creativity and Innovation, 1st Edition. Cambridge University Press; Gray. (2013). Free to Learn: Why Unleashing the Instinct to Play Will Make Our Children Happier, More Self-Reliant, and Better Students for Life. Basic Books.

12. Dennis (1970).

13. Graham (2010).

14. Baumeister et al. (2013). Some Key Differences Between a Happy Life and a Meaningful Life. The Journal of Positive Psychology, 8 (6), 505-516.

15. Csikszentmihalyi (2008). The Psychology of Optimal Experience. Harper Perennial Modern Classics.

16. Ryan et al. (1997). Intrinsic Motivation and Exercise Adherence. International Journal of Sport Psychology. Vol. 28.

17. Woolley et al. (2016). Immediate Rewards Predict Adherence to Long-Term Goals. Personality and Social Psychology Bulletin, 43 (2), 151–62.

18. Graham (2010).

19. Gray (2009). The Biological Distinction Between Play and Contest, and Their Merging in Modern Games. Psychology Today. https://www.psychologytoday.com/blog/freedom-learn/200911/the-biological-distinction-between-play-and-contest-and-their-merging-in

20. Gray (2009).

21. Thelen and Smith (2006). Dynamic Systems Theories, from Handbook of Child Psychology, Theoretical Models of Human Development, Vol. 1, 6th ed., p. 286. Ed. William Damon, Richard M. Lerner. John Wiley & Sons.

22. Bateson (2013).

23. Feynman (1997). Surely You're Joking, Mr. Feynman. W.W. Norton.

24. Brussoni et al. (2012). Risky Play and Children's Safety: Balancing Priorities for Optimal Child Development. International Journal of Environmental Research and Public Health, 9(9), 3134–3148.

25. Gray (2011).

26. For examples, see Gray (2011); Haidt and Lukianoff (2018). The Coddling of The American Mind. Penguin Press; Skenazy (2010). Free Range Kids. Jossey-Bass.

27. Ibid.

28. For research on the general health of hunter-gatherers, see: Pontzer et al. (2018). Hunter-Gatherers as Models in Public Health. Obesity Reviews, 19(December), 24–35; O'Keefe, et al. (2011). Exercise Like a Hunter-Gatherer: A Prescription for Organic Physical Fitness. Progress in Cardiovascular Diseases, May-Jun; 53(6):471-9; Raichlen et al. (2017). Physical Activity Patterns and Biomarkers of Cardiovascular Disease Risk in Hunter-Gatherers. American Journal of Human Biology, 29(2), 1–13; Lieberman (2013). The Story of The Human Body: Evolution, Health, and Disease. Vintage.

CHAPTER THREE: COMPLEXITY

1. For some good examples of expert and pundit fails in prediction, see Tetlock (2015). SuperForecasting: The Art and Science of Prediction. Random House.

2. An interesting article comparing neurons in a brain, voters in an election, and fish in a school: https://www.simonsfoundation.org/2018/06/19/schooling-fish-may-offer-insights-into-networked-neurons/

3. Ahn et al. (2006). The Limits of Reductionism in Medicine: Could Systems Biology Offer an Alternative? PLoS Medicine 3 (6), 709–13.

4. Ahn et al. (2006). The Clinical Applications of a Systems Approach. PLoS Medicine 3 (7), 956–60.

5. Plsek et al. (2010). Complexity Science: The Challenge of Complexity in Health Care. BMJ 323 (7313), 625–28.

6. For examples, see: Harbourne et al. (2009). Movement Variability and the Use of Nonlinear Tools: Principles to Guide Physical Therapist Practice. Physical Therapy 89 (3), 267–82; Thayer et al. (2012). A Meta-Analysis of Heart Rate Variability and Neuroimaging Studies: Implications for Heart Rate Variability as a Marker of Stress and Health. Neuroscience and Biobehavioral Reviews, 36(2), 747–756.

7. Johnson (2007). Simply Complexity: A Clear Guide to Complexity Theory. One World.

8. Johnson (2007).

9. Chapman et al. (2008.) Pain and Stress in a Systems Perspective: Reciprocal Neural, Endocrine, and Immune Interactions. The Journal of Pain: Official Journal of the American Pain Society 9 (2), 122–45.

10. Reichling et al. (2009). Critical Role of Nociceptor Plasticity in Chronic Pain. Trends in Neurosciences, 32(12), 611–18; Price et al. (2015). Commonalities Between Pain and Memory Mechanisms and Their Meaning for Understanding Chronic Pain. Progress in Molecular Biology and Translational Science, 131, 409–34.

11. This is Dan Dennett's "intentional stance," which he describes as follows: "First you decide to treat the object whose behavior is to be predicted as a rational agent; then you figure out what beliefs that agent ought to have, given its place in the world and its purpose. Then you figure out what desires it ought to have, on the same considerations, and finally you predict that this rational agent will act to further its goals in the light of its beliefs. A little practical reasoning from the chosen set of beliefs and desires will in most instances yield a decision about what the agent ought to do; that is what you predict the agent will do." For more on the intentional stance, see Dennett (1987). The

Intentional Stance. MIT Press. Or my blog post here: https://www.bettermovement.org/blog/2017/the-intentional-stance.

12. Meadows (1973). Thinking in Systems: A Primer. Chelsea Green Publishing.

13. Chapman et al. (2010). Painful Multi-Symptom Disorders, a Systems Perspective. Chapter One of Translational Pain Research: From Mouse to Man. Kruger and Light, editors. Taylor and Francis.

14. Ahn (2006); Plsek (2001).

15. Editorial, The Lancet (2018). UK Life Science Research: Time to Burst the Biomedical Bubble. The Lancet, 392 (10143), 187.

16. Meadows (1973); Chapman (2008).

17. Dobzhansky (1973). Nothing in Biology Makes Sense Except in the Light of Evolution. American Biology Teacher, 35 (3), 125–129.

18. Bittencourt et al. (2016). Complex Systems Approach for Sports Injuries: Moving from Risk Factor Identification to Injury Pattern Recognition—Narrative Review and New Concept. British Journal of Sports Medicine, 50(21), 1309–1314.

19. Harbourne (2009).

20. Chow, et al. (2015). Nonlinear Pedagogy in Skill Acquisition: An Introduction. 1st Edition, Routledge.

21. Hofstadter (1985). Metamagical Themas: Questing for the Essence of Mind and Pattern. Basic Books.

22. Taleb (2010). The Black Swan: The Impact of the Highly Improbable. Random House.

23. Chapman (2008).

24. Harbourne (2009).

25. Thayer (2012).

26. Thayer (2012); Grippo (2017). Opinion: Heart Rate Variability, Health and Well-Being: A Systems Perspective. Research Topic. Frontiers in Public Health, 5, 246.

27. Seely et al. (2004). Complex Systems and The Technology of Variability Analysis. Critical Care. 2004; 8(6): 367–R38; Moseley et al. (2006). Reduced Variability of Postural Strategy Prevents Normalization of Motor Changes Induced by Back Pain: A Risk Factor for Chronic Trouble? Behavioral Neuroscience, 120(2), 474–476.

28. Meadows (1973). Thinking in Systems: A Primer. Vermont. Chelsea Green Publishing.

29. Harbourne (2009).

30. Herzfeld et al. (2014). Motor Variability Is Not Noise, But Grist for The Learning Mill. Nature Neuroscience 17, 149-150; Wu et al. (2014). Temporal Structure of Motor Variability Is Dynamically Regulated and Predicts Motor Learning Ability. Nature Neuroscience 17, 312–321.

31. Thelen and Smith (2006). Dynamic Systems Theories, from Handbook of Child Psychology, Theoretical Models of Human Development, Vol. 1, 6th ed., p. 286. Ed. William Damon, Richard M. Lerner. John Wiley & Sons.

32. These landscapes are used in a wide variety of complex phenomena, including epigenetic cell development, ecological balance, and infant motor development.

33. Taleb (2010).

34. Von Foerster (1960). On Self-Organizing Systems and Their Environments, pp. 31–50 in Self-Organizing Systems. Ed. Yovits and Cameron. Pergamon Press; Prigogine and Stengers (1984). Order Out of Chaos: Man's New Dialogue with Nature. Bantam Books.

35. Taleb (2016). Antifragile: Things That Gain from Disorder. Random House; Gopnik (2016). The Gardener and the Carpenter: What the New Science of Child Development Tells Us About the Relationship Between Parents and Children. Farrar, Straus and Giroux; Gray, (2011). The Decline of Play and The Rise of Psychopathology in Children and Adolescents. American Journal of Play 3(4), 443–63; Jacobs (1961). The Death and Life of Great American Cities. Vintage Reissue Edition.

36. Bosch (2015). Strength Training and Coordination: An Integrative Approach. 2010 Publishers; Davids et al. (2012). Ecological Dynamics and Motor Learning Design in Sport. Skill Acquisition in Sport: Research, Theory and Practice. Chapter Seven of Skill Acquisition in Sport: Research, Theory & Practice, 2nd Ed., Editors: Williams and Hodges, Routledge; Glazier (2015). Towards a Grand Unified Theory of Sports Performance. Human Movement Science. Elsevier B.V., 1–18.

37. Glouberman et al. (2002). Complicated and Complex Systems: What Would Successful Reform of Medicare Look Like? Commission on Future of Health Care in Canada, Paper No. 8, (July), 1–37; Rickles, et al. (2007). A Simple Guide to Chaos and Complexity. Journal of Epidemiology and Community Health, 61(11), 933–937.

38. Glouberman (2002).

39. The Wikipedia entry on the KISS principle provides a good summary: https://en.wikipedia.org/wiki/KISS_principle

40. Plsek (2001). Redesigning Health Care with Insights from the Science of Complex Adaptive Systems. Appendix B to Crossing the Quality Chasm: A New Health System for the 21st Century. Institute of Medicine (US) Committee on Quality of Health Care in America.

41. A great quote from Friedrich Hayek: "If man is not to do more harm than good in his efforts to improve the social order, he will have to learn that in this, as in all other fields where essential complexity of an organized kind prevails, he cannot acquire the full knowledge which would make mastery of the events possible. He will therefore have to use what knowledge he can achieve, not to shape the results as the craftsman shapes his handiwork, but rather to cultivate a growth by providing the appropriate environment, in the manner in which the gardener does this for his plants." From: The Pretence of Knowledge, Nobel Memorial Lecture delivered in Stockholm (11 December 1974), reprinted as Ch. 2 of New Studies in Philosophy Politics, Economics and the History of Ideas (Routledge, 1978).

42. Gopnik (2016).

43. Meadows (1973).

44. Glazier (2015).

45. Kugler et al. (1980). On the Concept of Coordinative Structures as Dissipative Structures: Theoretical Lines of Convergence. Tutorials in Motor Behavior. Stelmach and Requin Eds. North Holland Publishing. Accessed from http://www.haskins.yale.edu/Reprints/HL0297.pdf

46. Davids et al. (2003). Acquiring Skill in Sport: A Constraints-Led Perspective. International Journal of Computer Science in Sport, 2 (2), 31-39.

47. Newell (1986). Constraints on The Development of Coordination Motor Development in Children: Aspects of Coordination and Control, 341–361. Editors: Wade and Whiting. Nijhoff.

48. Davids et al. (2012). Ecological Dynamics and Motor Learning Design in Sport. Skill Acquisition in Sport: Research, Theory and Practice. Chapter Seven of Skill Acquisition in Sport: Research, Theory & Practice, 2nd Ed. Editors: Williams and Hodges. Routledge.

CHAPTER FOUR: STRESS

1. McEwen (2007). Physiology and Neurobiology of Stress and Adaptation: Central Role of the Brain. Physiological Reviews, 87(3), 873–904.

2. Sapolsky (1994). Why Zebras Don't Get Ulcers. p. 22-23. Owl Books.

3. Ibid.

4. Ibid.

5. McEwen (2007).

6. Cohen (2007). Psychological Stress and Disease. JAMA, Oct 10, 298(14), 1685-7.

7. McEwen (2017). Neurobiological and Systemic Effects of Chronic Stress. Chronic Stress Volume 1, 1–11; McEwan (2007).

8. McEwen (2017); McEwan (2007).

9. Denver (2009. Structural and Functional Evolution of Vertebrate Neuroendocrine Stress Systems. Annals of the New York Academy of Science, 1163, 1–16.

10. Sapolsky (1994).

11. Ibid.

12. Sapolsky (1994); Brenner et al. (2015). Evolutionary Mismatch and Chronic Psychological Stress. Journal of Evolutionary Medicine, 3, 1–11; Lieberman (2013). The Story of the Human Body: Evolution, Health and Disease. Pantheon.

13. Sapolsky (1994).

14. McEwen (2007).

15. Moreno (2017). Variability and Practice Load in Motor Learning. Revista Internacional de Ciencias del Deporte, 11(39), 62-78.

16. Baechle and Earle (2000). Essentials of Strength Training and Conditioning, 2nd ed. Human Kinetics.

17. Lieberman (2015). Is Exercise Really Medicine? An Evolutionary Perspective. Current Sports Medicine Reports, 14(4), 313–319.

18. Gundersen (2016). Muscle Memory and A New Cellular Model for Muscle Atrophy and Hypertrophy. The Journal of Experimental Biology, 219 (2), 235-242.

19. Bonafiglia, et al. (2016). Inter-Individual Variability in the Adaptive Responses to Endurance and Sprint Interval Training: A Randomized Crossover Study. PloS one, 11(12), e0167790; For research on variability in response to strength training, see Ahtiainen, et al. (2016). Heterogeneity in Resistance Training-Induced Muscle Strength and Mass Responses in Men and Women of Different Ages. Journal of the American Aging Association, Feb;38(1), 10.

20. Xie et al. (2013). Sleep Drives Metabolite Clearance from The Adult Brain. Science. Oct 18; 342(6156), 373-7.

21. Kurina et al. (2013). Sleep Duration and All-Cause Mortality: A Critical Review of Measurement and Associations. Annals of Epidemiology, 23(6), 361–370.

22. Finan et al. (2013). The Association of Sleep and Pain: An Update and a Path Forward. The Journal of Pain, 14(12), 1539–1552.

23. Asih et al. (2014). Insomnia in a Chronic Musculoskeletal Pain with Disability Population Is Independent of Pain and Depression. Spine Journal, 14(9), 2000–2007; Choy (2015). The Role of Sleep in Pain and Fibromyalgia. Nature Reviews Rheumatology 11 (9), 513–20.

24. Simonelli et. al. (2019) Sleep Extension Reduces Pain Sensitivity. Sleep Medicine, 54, 172-176.

25. Fullagar et al. (2015). Sleep and Athletic Performance: The Effects of Sleep Loss on Exercise Performance, and Physiological and Cognitive Responses to Exercise. Sports Medicine, 45(2), 161–186.

26. Milewski et al. (2014). Chronic Lack of Sleep Is Associated with Increased Sports Injuries in Adolescent Athletes. Journal of Pediatric Orthopaedics, 34(2), 129–133.

27. Mah at al. (2011). The Effects of Sleep Extension on The Athletic Performance of Collegiate Basketball Players. Sleep, 34(7), 943-50.

28. McEwen 2007.

29. Ganzel et al. (2010). Allostasis and the Human Brain: Integrating Models of Stress from The Social and Life Sciences. Psychological Review 117(1), 134–74.

30. Vachon-Presseau, et al. (2013). Acute Stress Contributes to Individual Differences in Pain and Pain-Related Brain Activity in Healthy and Chronic Pain Patients. The Journal of Neuroscience, 33(16), 6826-6833; Ebrecht et al. (2004). Perceived Stress and Cortisol Levels Predict Speed of Wound Healing in Healthy Male Adults. Psychoneuroendocrinology. 29(6):798–809; Gouin et al. (2011). The Impact of Psychological Stress on Wound Healing: Methods and Mechanisms. Immunology and Allergy Clinics of North America. 31(1), 81–93.

31. McEwen 2007.

32. Mariotti (2015). The Effects of Chronic Stress on Health: New Insights into The Molecular Mechanisms of Brain-Body Communication. Future Science OA, 1(3), 23.

33. McEwen 2007.

34. Kiely (2016). A New Understanding of Stress and The Implications for Our Cultural Training Paradigm. New Studies in Athletics, 30:3; 27-35.

35. Bartholomew et al. (2008). Strength Gains After Resistance Training: The Effect of Stressful, Negative Life Events. Journal of Strength and Conditioning Research, 22(4), 1215–1221; Stults-Kolehmainen et al. (2014). Chronic Psychological Stress Impairs Recovery of Muscular Function and Somatic Sensations Over a 96-Hour Period. Journal of Strength and Conditioning Research, 28(7), 2007–2017; Walburn et al. (2009). Psychological Stress and Wound Healing in Humans: A Systematic Review and Meta-Analysis. Journal of Psychosomatic Research, 67(3), 253–271; Kiely (2016).

36. Geva et al. (2017). Triathletes Lose Their Advantageous Pain Modulation Under Acute Psychosocial Stress. Medicine and Science in Sports and Exercise, 49(2), 333–341.

37. Ivarsson et al. (2017). Psychosocial Factors and Sport injuries: Meta-Analyses for Prediction and Prevention. Sports Medicine 47, 353–65.

38. Li et al. (2017). Preseason Anxiety and Depressive Symptoms and Prospective Injury Risk in Collegiate Athletes. American Journal of Sports Medicine. 45(9), 2148-2155.

39. Saw et al. (2016). Monitoring the Athlete Training Response: Subjective Self-Reported Measures Trump Commonly Used Objective Measures: A Systematic Review. British Journal of Sports Medicine, 50(5), 281–291.

40. Kiely (2009). Periodization, Planning, Prediction: and Why the Future Ain't What It Used To Be! Techniques Journal of USA Track, Field and Cross-Country Association.

41. Bosch (2015). Strength Training and Coordination: An Integrative Approach. 2010 Publishers.

42. Brabban and Turkington (2002). The Search for Meaning: Detecting Congruence Between Life Events, Underlying Schema and Psychotic Symptoms. Chapter Five, a Casebook of Cognitive Therapy for Psychosis. Editor: Morrison.

43. Moseley and Butler (2015). The Explain Pain Handbook Protectometer, NOI Group.

44. Engle et al. (2008). Stress and The Neuroendocrine System: The Role of Exercise as a Stressor and Modifier of Stress. Expert Reviews in Endocrinology and Metabolism. 1(6): 783–792.

45. This is called the diathesis-stress model.

CHAPTER FIVE: FITNESS

1. Engle et al. (2008). Stress and The Neuroendocrine System: The Role of Exercise as a Stressor and Modifier of Stress. Expert Reviews in Endocrinology and Metabolism. 1(6): 783–792.

2. The Academy of Medical Royal Colleges (2015). Exercise: The Miracle Cure and The Role of The Doctor in Promoting It. Report from the Academy of Medical Royal Colleges, February.

3. Pedersen et al. (2015). Exercise as Medicine - Evidence for Prescribing Exercise as Therapy in 26 Different Chronic Diseases. Scandinavian Journal of Medicine and Science in Sports, 25, 1–72; Booth et al. (2012). Lack of Exercise Is a Major Cause of Chronic Diseases. Comprehensive Physiology, 2(2), 1143–1211; Piercy et al. (2018). The Physical Activity Guidelines for Americans. JAMA, 320(19), 2020.

4. For examples, see Foster et al. (2018). Prevention and Treatment of Low Back Pain: Evidence, Challenges, and Promising Directions. The Lancet, 391(10137), 2368–2383; Smith et al. (2014). An Update of Stabilisation Exercises For Low Back Pain: A Systematic Review With Meta-Analysis. BMC Musculoskeletal Disorders, 15(1); Ferreira (2007). Comparison of General Exercise, Motor Control Exercise and Spinal Manipulative Therapy for Chronic Low Back Pain: A Randomized Trial. Pain, 131(1–2), 31–37.

5. Bosomworth (2009). Exercise and Knee Osteoarthritis: Benefit or Hazard?" Canadian Family Physician 55(9), 871–78.

6. Pedersen (2015).

7. Pedersen (2015).

8. Erickson et al. (2011). Exercise Training Increases Size of Hippocampus and Improves Memory. Proceedings of the National Academy of Sciences of the United States of America 108(7), 3017–22.

9. Gomez-Pinilla et al. (2013). The Influence of Exercise on Cognitive Abilities. Comprehensive Physiology, 3(1), 403–28.

10. Nieman et al. (1999). Exercise and Immune Function. Recent Developments in Sports Medicine, 27(2), 73–80.

11. Pedersen (2015).

12. O'Donovan et al. (2017). Association of 'Weekend Warrior' and Other Leisure Time Physical Activity Patterns with Risks for All-Cause, Cardiovascular Disease, and Cancer Mortality. JAMA Internal Medicine, 175(6), 959–67.

13. NASA Information, Muscle Atrophy, accessed from https://www.nasa.gov/pdf/64249main_ffs_factsheets_hbp_atrophy.pdf. Interestingly, the reason for the bone loss doesn't seem to be related to lack of mechanical stress. The absence of gravity prevents the flow of liquid in the bone that signals the need for rebuilding.

14. Dittmer et al. (1993). Complications of Immobilization and Bed Rest. Part 1: Musculoskeletal and Cardiovascular Complications. Canadian Family Physician 39, 1428–32, 1435; Corcoran (1991). Use it Or Lose It--The Hazards

of Bed Rest and Inactivity. The Western Journal of Medicine 154(5), 536–38; Zarins (1982). Soft Tissue Injury and Repair--Biomechanical Aspects. International Journal of Sports Medicine 3, 9–11.

15. Piercy (2018); World Health Organisation. Global Recommendations on Physical Activity for Health. Geneva, 2010.

16. Lear et al. (2017). The Effect of Physical Activity on Mortality and Cardiovascular Disease in 130,000 People From 17 High-Income, Middle-Income, and Low-Income Countries: The PURE Study. The Lancet, 390(10113), 2643–2654.

17. Stamatakis, et al. (2017). Does Strength Promoting Exercise Confer Unique Health Benefits? A Pooled Analysis of Eleven Population Cohorts with All-Cause, Cancer, and Cardiovascular Mortality Endpoints. American Journal of Epidemiology, 187 (5), 1102-1112.

18. Piercy 2108.

19. For research on the general health of hunter-gatherers, see: Pontzer et al. (2018). Hunter-Gatherers as Models in Public Health. Obesity Reviews, 19(December), 24–35; O'Keefe, et al. (2011). Exercise Like a Hunter-Gatherer: A Prescription for Organic Physical Fitness. Progress in Cardiovascular Diseases. 53(6):471-9; Raichlen et al. (2017). Physical Activity Patterns and Biomarkers of Cardiovascular Disease Risk in Hunter-Gatherers. American Journal of Human Biology, 29(2), 1–13; Lieberman (2013). The Story of The Human Body: Evolution, Health, and Disease. Vintage.

20. Lieberman (2015). Is Exercise Really Medicine? An Evolutionary Perspective. Current Sports Medicine Reports, 14(4), 313–319.

21. Lieberman (2015); O'Keefe (2011).

22. Pontzer (2018); Raichlen (2017).

23. Lear (2017).

24. Pontzer (2018); O'Keefe (2011).

25. Iowa State University News Service (2017). High-intensity Workouts Send the Wrong Message, Says Iowa State Professor. https://www.news.iastate.edu/news/2017/10/03/hiit

26. Glazer, et al. (2013). Sustained and Shorter Bouts of Physical Activity Are Related To Cardiovascular Health. Medicine and Science in Sports and Exercise, 45(1), 109–115.

27. Gillen et al. (2014). Three Minutes of All-Out Intermittent Exercise Per Week Increases Skeletal Muscle Oxidative Capacity and Improves Cardiometabolic Health. PLoS One, 9, e111489.

28. Gillen et al. (2017). Twelve Weeks of Sprint Interval Training Improves Indices of Cardiometabolic Health Similar to Traditional Endurance Training Despite a Five-Fold Lower Exercise Volume and Time Commitment. PLoS One. 11(4), e0154075.

CHAPTER SIX: ENVIRONMENT

1. Munson (1993). Diseases of Captive Cheetahs (Acinonyx Jubatus): Results of the Cheetah Research Council Pathology Survey. Zoo Biology, 12(1), 105-124.

2. Haslam et al. (2018). Social Cure, What Social Cure? The Propensity to Underestimate the Importance of Social Factors for Health. Social Science & Medicine, Feb (198), 14-21. Adams et al. (2016). Why Are Some Population Interventions for Diet and Obesity More Equitable and Effective Than Others? The Role of Individual Agency. PLoS Medicine 13(4), e1001990.

3. Hajna et al. (2015). Associations between Neighbourhood Walkability and Daily Steps in Adults: A Systematic Review and Meta-Analysis. BMC Public Health 15 (1); Choi et al. (2017). Correlates Associated with Participation in Physical Activity Among Adults: A Systematic Review of Reviews and Update. BMC Public Health 17 (1), 356; Trost et al. (2002). Correlates of Adults' Participation in Physical Activity: Review and Update. Medicine and Science in Sports and Exercise. 34(12), 1996-2001.

4. Trost (2002).

5. Maas et al. (2006). Green Space, Urbanity, and Health: How Strong Is the Relation? Journal of Epidemiology and Community Health, 60(7), 587–592.

6. Ladwig et al. (2018). "My Best Memory Is When I Was Done with It": PE Memories Are Associated with Adult Sedentary Behavior. Translational Journal of the ACSM. 3(16), 119-129.

7. Christakis at al. (2007). The Spread of Obesity in a Large Social Network over 32 Years. New England Journal of Medicine. 357, 370-379.

8. Carrell et al. (2011). Is Poor Fitness Contagious?: Evidence from Randomly Assigned Friends. Journal of Public Economics. 95 (7–8), 657–63.

9. Thompson et al. (2011). Does Participating in Physical Activity in Outdoor Natural Environments Have a Greater Effect on Physical and Mental Wellbeing than Physical Activity Indoors? A Systematic Review. Environmental Science & Technology. 45(5), 1761–72.

10. Rogerson et al. (2016). Influences of Green Outdoors versus Indoors Environmental Settings on Psychological and Social Outcomes of Controlled Exercise. International Journal of Environmental Research and Public Health 13(4), 363.

11. Rogerson (2016).

12. "The perception that physical exertion serves some immediate purpose may be a key factor in determining affective response to exercise." Lee et al. (2016). The Exercise-Affect-Adherence Pathway: An Evolutionary Perspective. Frontiers in Psychology. 7, 1285.

13. Rogerson (2016).

14. Rogerson (2016).

15. Kuo (2015). How Might Contact with Nature Promote Human Health? Promising Mechanisms and a Possible Central Pathway. Frontiers in Psychology, 6(8), 1–8.

16. Ulrich (1984). View through a Window May Influence Recovery from Surgery. Science. 224 (4647), 420–21.

17. Alvarsson et al. (2010). Stress Recovery during Exposure to Nature Sound and Environmental Noise. International Journal of Environmental Research and Public Health 7(3), 1036–46; Kuo (2015).

18. Rietveld et al. (2014). A Rich Landscape of Affordances. Ecological Psychology 26(4), 325–52.

19. Fagereng (2010). A Real Game Examination of Visual Perception in Soccer. Unpublished Masters Thesis.

20. Lowe (2011). I'm a Romantic, says Xavi, Heartbeat of Barcelona and Spain. The Guardian. https://www.theguardian.com/football/2011/feb/11/xavi-barcelona-spain-interview

21. See Rafe's website Evolve Move Play. https://www.evolvemoveplay.com/

CHAPTER SEVEN: STRUCTURE

1. From an article at On Target Publications called Stuart McGill: Hip Anatomy. Accessed from https://www.otp-books.com/stuart-mcgill-hip-anatomy/

2. Trappe et al. (2015). Skeletal Muscle Signature of a Champion Sprint Runner. Journal of Applied Physiology, 118(12), 1460–1466.

3. Costill et al. (1976). Muscle Fiber Composition and Enzyme Activities of Elite Distance Runners. Medicine and Science in Sports, 8(2), 96–100.

4. Thelen and Smith (1994). A Dynamic Systems Approach to the Development of Cognition and Action. The MIT Press.

5. Schoenfeld (2010). The Mechanisms of Muscle Hypertrophy and Their Application to Resistance Training. Journal of Strength and Conditioning Research 24(10), 2857–72.

6. Khan et al. (2009). Mechanotherapy: How Physical Therapists' Prescription of Exercise Promotes Tissue Repair. British Journal of Sports Medicine 43(4), 247–52.

7. Chan et al. (2006). Genetics of Disc Degeneration. European Spine Journal, 15(3), 317-25.

8. Belavý et al. (2017). Running Exercise Strengthens the Intervertebral Disc. Scientific Reports. 7, 45975.

9. Bosomworth (2009). Exercise and Knee Osteoarthritis: Benefit or Hazard? Canadian Family Physician 55(9), 871–78; Chakravarty et al. (2008). Long Distance Running and Knee Osteoarthritis. A Prospective Study. American Journal of Preventive Medicine. 35(2), 133–38; Lo et al. (2017). Is There an Association Between a History of Run-

ning and Symptomatic Knee Osteoarthritis? A Cross-Sectional Study from The Osteoarthritis Initiative. Arthritis Care & Research 69(2), 183–91.

10. Wallace et al. (2017). Knee Osteoarthritis Has Doubled in Prevalence Since the Mid-20th Century. Proceedings of the National Academy of Sciences of the United States of America 114 (35), 9332–36.

11. Dimock et al. (2017). Compensating for Loss: Running on One Tibialis Anterior. BMJ Case Reports 2017. (May), 19834.

12. Personal communication.

13. Jensen et al. (1994). Magnetic Resonance Imaging of The Lumbar Spine in People Without Back Pain. New England Journal of Medicine 331(2), 69–73.

14. Boden et al. (1990). Abnormal Magnetic-Resonance Scans of The Lumbar Spine in Asymptomatic Subjects. A Prospective Investigation. The Journal of Bone and Joint Surgery. American Volume 72(3), 403–8.

15. Nakashima et al. (2015). Abnormal Findings on Magnetic Resonance Images of The Cervical Spines in 1211 Asymptomatic Subjects. Spine 40(6), 392–98.

16. Brinjikji et al. (2015). MRI Findings of Disc Degeneration Are More Prevalent in Adults with Low Back Pain Than in Asymptomatic Controls: A Systematic Review and Meta-Analysis. American Journal of Neuroradiology 36 (12).

17. Borenstein et al. (2001). The Value of Magnetic Resonance Imaging of The Lumbar Spine to Predict Low-Back Pain in Asymptomatic Subjects: A Seven-Year Follow-Up Study. The Journal of Bone and Joint Surgery. American Volume 83–A(9), 1306–11.

18. Tonosu et al. (2017). The Associations Between Magnetic Resonance Imaging Findings and Low Back Pain: A 10-Year Longitudinal Analysis. PLoS One. 12(11), e0188057.

19. Silvis et al. (2011). High Prevalence of Pelvic and Hip Magnetic Resonance Imaging Findings in Asymptomatic Collegiate and Professional Hockey Players. The American Journal of Sports Medicine 39(4), 715–21.

20. Beattie et al. (2005). Abnormalities Identified in The Knees of Asymptomatic Volunteers Using Peripheral Magnetic Resonance Imaging. Osteoarthritis and Cartilage 13(3), 181–86.

21. Tempelhof et al. (1999). Age-Related Prevalence of Rotator Cuff Tears in Asymptomatic Shoulders. Journal of Shoulder and Elbow Surgery. 8(4), 296–99.

22. Connor et al. (2003). Magnetic Resonance Imaging of the Asymptomatic Shoulder of Overhead Athletes. The American Journal of Sports Medicine 31(5), 724–27.

23. Kolata (2011). Sports Medicine Said to Overuse M.R.I.'S. New York Times. Accessed from https://www.nytimes.com/2011/10/29/health/mris-often-overused-often-mislead-doctors-warn.html

24. Wáng et al. (2018). Informed Appropriate Imaging for Low Back Pain Management: A Narrative Review. Journal of Orthopaedic Translation, 15(August), 21–34.

25. Webster et al. (2010). Relationship of Early Magnetic Resonance Imaging for Work-Related Acute Low Back Pain with Disability and Medical Utilization Outcomes. Journal of Occupational and Environmental Medicine. 52(9), 900–907; Webster et al. (2013). Iatrogenic Consequences of Early Magnetic Resonance Imaging in Acute, Work-Related, Disabling Low Back Pain. Spine. 38(22), 1939-46.

26. Culvenor et al. (2018). Prevalence of Knee Osteoarthritis Features On Magnetic Resonance Imaging In Asymptomatic Uninjured Adults: A Systematic Review And Meta-Analysis. British Journal of Sports Medicine. bjsports-2018-099257.

27. Heidari, et al. (2011). Knee Osteoarthritis Prevalence, Risk Factors, Pathogenesis and Features: Part I. Caspian Journal of Internal Medicine 2(2), 205–12.

28. Lubowitz (2002). A Controlled Trial of Arthroscopic Surgery for Osteoarthritis of The Knee. Arthroscopy 18(8), 950–51.

29. Kolata (2013). Why 'Useless' Surgery Is Still Popular. New York Times. http://www.nytimes.com/2016/08/04/upshot/the-right-to-know-that-an-operation-is-next-to-useless.html?_r=2

30. Kirkely et al. (2008). A Randomized Trial of Arthroscopic Surgery for Osteoarthritis of The Knee. New England Journal. 359, 1097.

31. Thorlund, et al. (2015). Arthroscopic Surgery for Degenerative Knee: Systematic Review and Meta-Analysis of Benefits and Harms. British Medical Journal. 350 (3), 2747–2747.

32. Brignardello-Petersen et al. (2017). Knee Arthroscopy Versus Conservative Management in Patients with Degenerative Knee Disease: A Systematic Review. BMJ Open 7(5), e016114; Sihvonen et al. (2017). Arthroscopic Partial Meniscectomy Versus Placebo Surgery for a Degenerative Meniscus Tear: A 2-Year Follow-Up of the Randomised Controlled Trial. Annals of the Rheumatic Diseases. 77(2), 188-195.

33. Järvinen et al. (2016). Arthroscopic Surgery for Knee Pain. BMJ (Clinical Research Ed.) 354 (July), i3934.

34. Siemieniuk et al. (2017). Arthroscopic Surgery for Degenerative Knee Arthritis and Meniscal Tears: A Clinical Practice Guideline. BMJ, j1982.

35. Jarvinen (2016).

36. Diamond et al. (2003). Management of Acute Osteoporotic Vertebral Fractures: A Nonrandomized Trial Comparing Percutaneous Vertebroplasty With Conservative Therapy. The American Journal of Medicine 114(4), 257–65.

37. Kallmes et al. (2009). A Randomized Trial of Vertebroplasty for Osteoporotic Spinal Fractures. New England Journal of Medicine 361(6), 569–79.

38. Mannion et al. (2013). Comparison of Spinal Fusion and Nonoperative Treatment in Patients with Chronic Low Back Pain: Long-Term Follow-Up of Three Randomized Controlled Trials. The Spine Journal. 13(11), 1438–48.

39. Saltychev, et al. (2014). Lumbar Fusion Compared with Conservative Treatment in Patients with Chronic Low Back Pain. International Journal of Rehabilitation Research 37(1), 2–8.

40. Bogduk et al. (2009). Is Spinal Surgery Effective for Back Pain? F1000 Medicine Reports 1 (July), 27–29.

41. Jain et al. (2014). Epidemiology of Musculoskeletal Upper Extremity Ambulatory Surgery in The United States. BMC Musculoskeletal Disorders 15(1), 4.

42. Steuri et al. (2017). Effectiveness of Conservative Interventions Including Exercise, Manual Therapy and Medical Management in Adults with Shoulder Impingement: A Systematic Review and Meta-Analysis of RCTs. British Journal of Sports Medicine. bjsports-2016-096515.

43. Ketola et al. (2013). No Evidence of Long-Term Benefits of Arthroscopicacromioplasty in The Treatment of Shoulder Impingement Syndrome: Five-Year Results of a Randomised Controlled Trial. Bone and Joint Research 2(7), 132–39.

44. Brox et al. (2017). Author Response—Sham Surgery Versus Labral Repair or Biceps Tenodesis for Type II Slap Lesions of The Shoulder: A Three-Armed Randomised Clinical Trial. British Journal of Sports Medicine, bjsports-2017-098251.

45. McElvany et al. (2015). Rotator Cuff Repair. The American Journal of Sports Medicine 43(2), 491–500.

46. According to Dr. Lawrence Gullotta, "When your rotator cuff is torn, you attribute all your pain and dysfunction to your torn rotator cuff, then you have it fixed and you feel better, but sometimes when you take an ultrasound or an MRI, the rotator cuff looks exactly like it did before you had the surgery." From this article: Large Study of Arthroscopic Rotator Cuff Repair Reveals Some Surprises. http://www.hss.edu/newsroom_study-arthroscopic-rotator-cuff-repair-surprises.asp

47. Beard et al. (2017). Arthroscopic Subacromial Decompression for Subacromial Shoulder Pain (Csaw): A Multicentre, Pragmatic, Parallel Group, Placebo-Controlled, Three-Group, Randomised Surgical Trial. The Lancet. 391, 329–38.

48. Schreurs et al. (2017). No Benefit of Arthroscopy in Subacromial Shoulder Pain. The Lancet. 6736 (17).

49. Threlkeld (1992). The Effects of Manual Therapy on Connective Tissue. Physical Therapy. 72(12), 893–902; Chaudry, Schleip (2008). Three-Dimensional Mathematical Model for Deformation of Human Fasciae in Manual Therapy. Journal of American Osteopathic Association. 8(108), 379–390.

50. Schleip (2003). Fascial Plasticity – A New Neurobiological Explanation: Part 1. J Bodywork and Movement Therapies. 7(1), 11–9.

51. Cramer et al. (2012). Quantification of Cavitation and Gapping of Lumbar Zygapophyseal Joints During Spinal Manipulative Therapy. Journal of Manipulative and Physiological Therapeutics. 35(8), 614–21.

52. Shilton et al. (2015). Does Cervical Lordosis Change After Spinal Manipulation for Non-Specific Neck Pain? A Prospective Cohort Study. Chiropractic & Manual Therapies 23, 33; Tullberg (1998). Manipulation Does Not Alter the Position of the Sacroiliac Joint. A Roentgen Stereophotogrammetric Analysis. Spine. 23(10), 1124–1129.

53.   Ross et al. (2004). Determining Cavitation Location During Lumbar and Thoracic Spinal Manipulation: Is Spinal Manipulation Accurate and Specific? Spine. 29(13),1452–7.

54.   Bialosky et al. (2012). Basis for Spinal Manipulative Therapy: A Physical Therapist Perspective. Journal of Electromyography and Kinesiology: Official Journal of the International Society of Electrophysiological Kinesiology. 22(5), 643–47.

55.   Flynn et al. (2003). The Audible Pop Is Not Necessary for Successful Spinal High-Velocity Thrust Manipulation in Individuals with Low Back Pain. Archives of Physical Medical Rehabilitation. 84(7), 1057–60.

56.   Gross et al. (2010). Manipulation or Mobilisation for Neck Pain: A Cochrane Review. Manual Therapy. 15(4), 315-33; Schomacher (2009). The Effect of An Analgesic Mobilization Technique When Applied at Symptomatic or Asymptomatic Levels of The Cervical Spine in Subjects with Neck Pain: A Randomized Controlled Trial. The Journal of Manual & Manipulative Therapy. 17(2), 101–108.

57.   Bialosky et al. (2009). The Mechanisms of Manual Therapy in The Treatment of Musculoskeletal Pain: A Comprehensive Model. Manual Therapy. 14(5), 531–8.

58   I am not addressing here the issue of trigger points, which are a controversial issue. See, for example, this article from Paul Ingraham: https://www.painscience.com/articles/trigger-point-doubts.php

59.   Vasseljen et al. (1996). Can Stress-Related Shoulder and Neck Pain Develop Independently of Muscle Activity? Pain 64(2), 221–30; Maigne et al. (2012). Lower Back Pain and Neck Pain: Is It Possible to Identify the Painful Side by Palpation Only? Annals of Physical and Rehabilitation Medicine 55(2), 103–11.

60.   Andersen et al. (2010). Increased Trapezius Pain Sensitivity Is Not Associated with Increased Tissue Hardness. The Journal of Pain. 11(5), 491–99.

61.   Paley (2016). Tibial Hemimelia: New Classification and Reconstructive Options. Journal of Children's Orthopaedics. 10(6), 529-555.

62.   Lauersen (2018). Strength Training as Superior, Dose-Dependent and Safe Prevention of Acute and Overuse Sports Injuries: A Systematic Review, Qualitative Analysis and Meta-Analysis. British Journal of Sports Medicine. 52(24), 1557-1563.

63.   Longman (1996). Lewis Thinks Gold and Pumps Iron. New York Times. https://www.nytimes.com/1996/02/05/sports/lewis-thinks-gold-and-pumps-iron.html

64.   Balsalobre-Fernández et al. (2016). Effects of Strength Training on Running Economy in Highly Trained Runners. Journal of Strength and Conditioning Research. 30(8), 2361–68.

65.   Foster et al. (2007). Running Economy: The Forgotten Factor in Elite Performance. Sports Medicine 37(4–5), 316–19.

66.   Evening Standard. Mo-tivator: How Mo Farah's Coach Trained Him Up for a Double Olympic Gold Success. https://www.standard.co.uk/olympics/olympic-news/mo-tivator-how-mo-farahs-coach-trained-him-up-for-a-double-olympic-gold-success-8038354.html

CHAPTER EIGHT: MOBILITY

1.   Castori (2012) Ehlers-Danlos Syndrome, Hypermobility Type: An Underdiagnosed Hereditary Connective Tissue Disorder with Mucocutaneous, Articular, And Systemic Manifestations. ISRN Dermatology. 2012, 751768.

2.   Trehearn et al. (2009). Sit-and-Reach Flexibility and Running Economy of Men and Women Collegiate Distance Runners. Journal of Strength and Conditioning Research. 23(1), 158-62;

3.   Freckleton et al. (2013) Risk Factors for Hamstring Muscle Strain Injury in Sport: A Systematic Review and Meta-Analysis. British Journal of Sports Medicine 47(6), 351–58; Tyler et al. (2010). Groin Injuries in Sports Medicine. Sports Health. 2(3), 231–236.

4.   Sedaghati et al. (2013). Review of Sport-Induced Groin Injuries. Trauma Monthly. 18(3), 107–112; Behm et al. (2016). Acute Effects of Muscle Stretching on Physical Performance, Range of Motion, And Injury Incidence in Healthy Active Individuals: A Systematic Review. Applied Physiology. Nutrition, and Metabolism. 41(1), 1–11.

5.   Hart (2005). Effect of Stretching on Sport Injury Risk: A Review. Clinical Journal of Sport Medicine: Official Journal of the Canadian Academy of Sport Medicine. 15(2), 113.

6.   Al Attar, et al. (2017). Effect of Injury Prevention Programs That Include the Nordic Hamstring Exercise on Ham-
     string Injury Rates in Soccer Players: A Systematic Review And Meta-Analysis. Sports Medicine. 47(5), 907–916.

7.   Harøy et al. (2018). The Adductor Strengthening Programme Prevents Groin Problems Among Male Football
     Players: A Cluster-Randomised Controlled Trial. British Journal of Sports Medicine, 1–8; Tyler (2010).

8.   Strength training is also an effective way to prevent other overuse and acute injuries, reducing risk by 30-50%.
     Laursen et al. (2014). The Effectiveness of Exercise Interventions To Prevent Sports Injuries: A Systematic Review
     And Meta-Analysis Of Randomised Controlled Trials. British Journal of Sports Medicine. 48(11), 871-7.

9.   Williams (1990). Use of Intermittent Stretch in The Prevention of Serial Sarcomere Loss in Immobilised Muscle.
     Annals of the Rheumatic Diseases. 49(5), 316–317.

10. Harris et al. (2016). Radiographic Prevalence of Dysplasia, Cam, And Pincer Deformities in Elite Ballet. The
     American Journal of Sports Medicine. 44(1), 20–27.

11. Weppler et al. (2010). Increasing Muscle Extensibility: A Matter of Increasing Length or Modifying Sensation?
     Physical Therapy. 90 (3): 438–49.

12. Zedka et al. (1999). Voluntary and Reflex Control of Human Back Muscles During Induced Pain. The Journal of
     Physiology. 520(2), 591-604.

13. The common explanation for frozen shoulder is structural – connective tissues in the joint become contracted and
     fibrotic. But it appears that muscle guarding due to pain may be the more important limiting factor in many cases.
     See Hollmann et al. (2018). Does Muscle Guarding Play A Role in Range Of Motion Loss In Patients With Frozen
     Shoulder? Musculoskeletal Science and Practice. 10(37), 64-68

CHAPTER NINE: POSTURE

1.   Posture is defined in various ways. I like the definition provided by Nicolai Bernstein, which focuses on the organi-
     zation of the trunk and neck. See Bernstein (1996). Dexterity and Its Development. Edited by Latash, Turvey and
     Lawrence. Routledge.

2.   Ivanenko and Gurfinkel (2018). Human Postural Control. Frontiers in Neuroscience. 12, 171.

3.   Gruters et al. (2017). The Eardrums Move When the Eyes Move: A Multisensory Effect on the Mechanics of Hear-
     ing. Proceedings of the National Academy of Sciences. 115(6), 1309-1318.

4.   Chagnaud et al. (2015). Spinal Corollary Discharge Modulates Motion Sensing During Vertebrate Locomotion.
     Nature Communications. 6, 7982.

5.   Bernstein (1996). "Usually, [the postural system] justifies our confidence, does not like interference in its business,
     and carries on its duty as reliably as the internal body organs. For example, the duodenum and the spleen also
     rarely report their work to consciousness!"

6.   Grundy et al. (1984). Does Unequal Leg Length Cause Back Pain? A Case-Control Study. The Lancet. 2(8397),
     256–58.

7.   Pope et al. (1985). The Relationship between Anthropometric, Postural, Muscular, and Mobility Characteristics of
     Males Ages 18-55. Spine 10(7), 644–48.

8.   Grob et al. (2007). The Association between Cervical Spine Curvature and Neck Pain. European Spine Journal
     16(5), 669–78.

9.   Nourbakhsh et al. (2002). Relationship between Mechanical Factors and Incidence of Low Back Pain. The Journal
     of Orthopaedic and Sports Physical Therapy. 32(9), 447–60.

10. Dieck et al. (1985). An Epidemiologic Study of the Relationship between Postural Asymmetry in the Teen Years
     and Subsequent Back and Neck Pain. Spine 10(10), 872–77.

11. Franklin et al. (1998). An Analysis of Posture and Back Pain in the First and Third Trimesters of Pregnancy. Jour-
     nal of Orthopaedic & Sports Physical Therapy 28(3), 133–38.

12. Barrett et al. (2016). Is Thoracic Spine Posture Associated with Shoulder Pain, Range of Motion and Function? A
     Systematic Review. Manual Therapy. 26(December), 38–46.

13. Richards et al. (2016). Neck Posture Clusters and Their Association With Biopsychosocial Factors and Neck Pain in Australian Adolescents. Physical Therapy 96(10), 1576–87.

14. Andrade et al. (2015). Systematic Review of Observational Studies Reveals No Association between Low Back Pain and Lumbar Spondylolysis with or without Isthmic Spondylolisthesis. European Spine Journal. 24(6), 1289–95.

15. Ettinger et al. (1994). Kyphosis in Older Women and Its Relation to Back Pain, Disability and Osteopenia: The Study of Osteoporotic Fractures. Osteoporosis International. 4(1), 55–60.

16. Damasceno et al. (2018). Text Neck and Neck Pain in 18–21-Year-Old Young Adults. European Spine Journal. 27 (6).

17. Campos et al. (2018). Exercise Programs May Be Effective in Preventing a New Episode of Neck Pain: A Systematic Review and Meta-Analysis. Journal of Physiotherapy. 64 (3), 159–65.

18. Chaléat-Valayer et al. (2011). Sagittal Spino-Pelvic Alignment in Chronic Low Back Pain. European Spine Journal. 20(s5), 634–40; Smith et al. (2008). Classification of Sagittal Thoraco-Lumbo-Pelvic Alignment of the Adolescent Spine in Standing and Its Relationship to Low Back Pain. Spine. 33(19), 2101–7.

19. Christensen et al. (2008). Spinal Curves and Health: A Systematic Critical Review of the Epidemiological Literature Dealing With Associations Between Sagittal Spinal Curves and Health. Journal of Manipulative and Physiological Therapeutics. 31(9), 690–714.

20. Théroux et al. (2015). Prevalence and Management of Back Pain in Adolescent Idiopathic Scoliosis Patients: A Retrospective Study. Pain Research & Management: The Journal of the Canadian Pain Society. 20(3), 153–57.

21. Hartvigsen et al. (2002). Does Sitting at Work Cause Low Back Pain? Ugeskrift for Laeger. 164(6), 759–61.

22. Wai et al. (2010). Causal Assessment of Occupational Lifting and Low Back Pain: Results of a Systematic Review. The Spine Journal. 10 (6), 554–66.

23. Kwon (2011). Systematic Review: Occupational Physical Activity and Low Back Pain. Occupational Medicine 61(8), 541–48.

24. Waddell et al. (2001). Occupational Health Guide Lines for The Management Of Low Back Pain At Work: Evidence Review. Occupational Medicine. 51(2), 124-135.

25. Shiri et al. (2010). The Association between Smoking and Low Back Pain: A Meta-Analysis. The American Journal of Medicine. 123(1), 87; Hoogendoorn et al. (2000). Systematic Review of Psychosocial Factors at Work and Private Life as Risk Factors for Back Pain. Spine 25(16), 2114–25.

26. Hodges et al. (2003). Experimental Muscle Pain Changes Feedforward Postural Responses of the Trunk Muscles. Experimental Brain Research. 151(2), 262–71.

27. Lederman (2007). The Myth of Core Stability. CPDO, 1–17; White et al. (2002). Abdominal and Erector Spinae Muscle Activity During Gait: The Use Of Cluster Analysis To Identify Patterns Of Activity. Clinical Biomechanics. 17(3), 177- 84.

28. Smith et al. (2014). An Update of Stabilisation Exercises for Low Back Pain: A Systematic Review with Meta-Analysis. BMC Musculoskeletal Disorders. 15 (1); Lederman (2007); Middelkoop (2010). Exercise Therapy for Chronic Nonspecific Low-Back Pain. Best Practice & Research Clinical Rheumatology 24 (2), 193–204.

29. O'Sullivan et al. (2018). Cognitive Functional Therapy: An Integrated Behavioral Approach for the Targeted Management of Disabling Low Back Pain. Physical Therapy. 98 (5), 408–23; See also Brumagne et al. (2008). Persons With Recurrent Low Back Pain Exhibit A Rigid Postural Control Strategy. European Spine Journal. 17(9), 1177-84; Claeys, et al. (2010). Decreased Variability In Postural Control Strategies In Young People With Non-Specific Low Back Pain Is Associated With Altered Proprioceptive Reweighting. European Journal of Applied Physiology. 111(1), 115-23.

30. Hodges (2011). Moving Differently In Pain: A New Theory To Explain The Adaptation To Pain. Pain. 152(3 Suppl), S90–8.

31. Mannion et al. (2012). Spine Stabilisation Exercises in the Treatment of Chronic Low Back Pain: A Good Clinical Outcome Is Not Associated with Improved Abdominal Muscle Function. European Spine Journal. 21(7), 1301–10; Steiger et al. (2012). Is a Positive Clinical Outcome after Exercise Therapy for Chronic Non-Specific Low Back Pain Contingent upon a Corresponding Improvement in the Targeted Aspect(s) of Performance? A Systematic Review. European Spine Journal. 21(4): 575–98.

32.   Moseley et al. (2006). Reduced Variability of Postural Strategy Prevents Normalization of Motor Changes Induced
      by Back Pain: A Risk Factor for Chronic Trouble? Behavioral Neuroscience. 120(2), 474–76.

CHAPTER TEN: SKILL

1.   Bernstein (1996). Dexterity and Its Development. Edited by Latash, Turvey and Lawrence. Routledge; Shum-
      way-Cook et al. (2012). Motor Control, 4th Edition, p. 12-14. Lippincott, Williams and Wilkins.
2.   Bernstein (1996).
3.   Bernstein (1967). The Coordination and Regulation of Movements. Pergamon Press.
4.   Latash (2012). The Bliss (Not the Problem) of Motor Abundance (not Redundancy). Experimental Brain Research.
      217(1), 1–5.
5.   Latash (2012); Harbourne et al. (2009). Movement Variability and the Use of Nonlinear Tools: Principles to Guide
      Physical Therapist Practice. Physical Therapy. 89(3), 267–282.
6.   Bernstein (1996).
7.   Shumway-Cook (2012) at 31; Bernstein (1996) at 411-413; Vereijken et al. (1992). Freezing Degrees of Freedom in
      Skill Acquisition. Journal of Motor Behavior. 24(1), 133–142.
8.   Shumway-Cook (2012 at 31 citing Broderick et al. (1999). Coordination Patterns in Ball Bouncing as a Function
      of Skill. Journal of Motor Behavior. 31(2), 165–188.
9.   Bernstein (1996) at 411-413.
10.   Shumway (2012) at 31. citing Southard et al. (1987). Changing Movement Patterns: Effects of Demonstration and
      Practice. Research Quarterly for Exercise and Sport. 58(1), 77–80.
11.   Shumway-Cook (2012) at 31.
12.   Bernstein (1996) at 115. Bernstein called these levels A, B, C and D but I have used numbers for clarity. He also
      divided his levels into sub levels, so the discussion here provides far less detail.
13.   Although Bernstein's work in this area is rather original and speculative, it continues to draw serious consideration
      from leading experts in motor control. See Profeta et al. (2018). Bernstein's Levels of Movement Construction: A
      Contemporary Perspective. Human Movement Science. 57, 111–33; Chow et al. (2015). Nonlinear Pedagogy in
      Skill Acquisition: An Introduction, p. 121. Routledge
14.   Bernstein (1996) at 120.
15.   Bernstein (1996) at 121-130.
16.   Marder et al. (2001). Central Pattern Generators and the Control of Rhythmic Movements. Current Biology: CB
      11 (23), 986-96; Guertin (2009). The Mammalian Central Pattern Generator for Locomotion. Brain Research Re-
      views. 62 (1), 45–56.
17.   Profeta et al. (2018).
18.   Schücker et al. (2018). Thinking about Your Running Movement Makes You Less Efficient: Attentional Focus
      Effects on Running Economy And Kinematics. Journal of Sports Sciences. 1–9.
19.   McBeath et al. (1995). How Baseball Outfielders Determine Where to Run to Catch Fly Balls. Science. 268(5210),
      569-573.
20.   Shaffer et al. (2004). How Dogs Navigate to Catch Frisbees. Psychological Science. 15(7), 437–41.
21.   Thelen and Smith (2006). Dynamic Systems Theories, p. 286. In Handbook of Child Psychology, Theoretical Mod-
      els of Human Development, Vol. 1, 6th ed. Damon, Lerner eds. John Wiley & Sons.
22.   Glazier et al. (2003). Dynamical Systems Theory: A Relevant Framework For Performance-Oriented Sports Bio-
      mechanics Research. SportScience. 7(1997), 1–8.
23.   Hamacher et al. (2018). Development of Functional Variability during the Motor Learning Process of a Complex
      Cyclic Movement. Journal of Biomechanics. 77, 124–30.
24.   Schmidt and Lee (2005). Motor Control and Learning: A Behavioral Emphasis. p. 193. Human Kinetics.
25.   Bosch (2015). Strength Training and Coordination: An Integrative Approach. 2010 Publishers.
26.   Coaches can consciously discover the fundamentals for a given activity by observing how the best performers
      move, noting similarities and differences. For example, pro tennis players use many different grips, rhythms, swing

trajectories and footwork patterns in hitting forehands, but there is a non-trivial list of fundamentals that all pros observe on every stroke. It is not easy to determine which aspects of good form are universal or contingent, and coaches will disagree on this subject. In fact, many of the "rules" for good movement proposed by experts are violated by top athletes on a regular basis. (See later in the chapter for some examples related to running.)

27. Yao et al. (2009). Variable Practice Versus Constant Practice in the Acquisition of Wheelchair Propulsive Speeds. Perceptual and Motor Skills. 109(1), 133–39; Ranganathan et al. (2013). Changing Up the Routine. Exercise and Sport Sciences Reviews. 41(1), 64–70.

28. Herzfeld et al. (2014). Motor Variability Is Not Noise, but Grist for the Learning Mill. Nature Neuroscience. 17(2), 149-50; Wu et al. (2014). Temporal Structure of Motor Variability Is Dynamically Regulated and Predicts Motor Learning Ability. Nature Neuroscience 17(2), 312–321.

29. Kirsh et al. (1994). On Distinguishing Epistemic from Pragmatic Action. Cognitive Science. 18, 513-549.

30. This is an example of "embodied cognition." Information is stored in certain positions or movements of the body, so the brain doesn't have to work as hard in representing that information. This is similar to how we keep track of a number while counting, by changing how many fingers we are holding up.

31. Wulf (2007). Attention and Motor Skill Learning. Human Kinetics. For a good summary of her research, see Benz et al. (2016). Coaching Instructions and Cues for Enhancing Sprint Performance. Strength and Conditioning Journal. 38, 1–11.

32. Porter et al. (2010). Focus of Attention and Verbal Instructions: Strategies of Elite Track and Field Coaches and Athletes. Sport Science Review. XIX: 199–211.

33. Benz (2016).

34. Benz (2016).

35. McKay et al. (2012). A Distal External Focus Enhances Novice Dart Throwing Performance. International Journal of Sport, Exercise and Psychology. 10, 149–156.

36. Wulf et al. (2007). An External Focus of Attention Enhances Golf Shot Accuracy In Beginners And Experts. Research Questions in Exercise and Sport. 78, 384–389.

37. Benz (2016).

38. Wulf et al. (1998). Instructions for Motor Learning: Differential Effects of Internal Versus External Focus Of Attention. Journal of Motor Behavior. 30, 169–179.

39. Wulf et al. (2001). The Automaticity of Complex Motor Skill Learning As A Function Of Attentional Focus. Quarterly Journal of Experimental Psychology Section A: Human Experimental Psychology. 54, 1143–1154.

40. Glazier (2015). Towards a Grand Unified Theory of Sports Performance. Human Movement Science. Elsevier B.V., 1–18; Gray (2011). Links Between Attention, Performance Pressure, and Movement in Skilled Motor Action. Current Directions in Psychological Science 20(5), 301–6.

41. Glazier (2015); Masters (1992). Knowledge, Knerves and Know-how: The Role Of Explicit Versus Implicit Knowledge In The Breakdown Of A Complex Motor Skill Under Pressure. British Journal of Psychology. 83, 343–358.

42. Sahrmann (2001) Diagnosis and Treatment of Movement Systems Impairment Syndromes, 1st Ed, p.3. Mosby.

43. Tumminello, Silvernail and Cormack (2017). The Corrective Exercise Trap. Personal Training Quarterly. 4(1), 6–15.

44. Lehman (2018). The Role and Value of Symptom-Modification Approaches in Musculoskeletal Practice. Journal of Orthopedic Sports and Physical Therapy. 48(6), 430-435.

45. Azevedo et al. (2018). Movement System Impairment-Based Classification Treatment Versus General Exercises for Chronic Low Back Pain: Randomized Controlled Trial. Physical Therapy. 98 (1), 28–39; Dillen et al. (2016). Efficacy of Classification-Specific Treatment and Adherence On Outcomes in People with Chronic Low Back Pain. A One-Year Follow-Up, Prospective, Randomized, Controlled Clinical Trial. Manual Therapy. 24, 52-64; Riley et al. (2018). Are Movement-Based Classification Systems More Effective Than Therapeutic Exercise or Guideline Based Care in Improving Outcomes for Patients with Chronic Low Back Pain? A Systematic Review. Journal of Manual & Manipulative Therapy. 1–10.

46. Saragiotto et al. (2016). Motor Control Exercise for Chronic Non-Specific Low-Back Pain. The Cochrane Database of Systematic Reviews. 8(1), CD012004.

47. Kim et al. (2014). Effects of External Pelvic Compression on Trunk and Hip Muscle EMG Activity During Prone Hip Extension in Females with Chronic Low Back Pain. Manual Therapy 19 (5), 467–71; Lehman (2006). Trunk and Hip Muscle Recruitment Patterns during the Prone Leg Extension Following a Lateral Ankle Sprain: A Prospective Case Study Pre and Post Injury. Chiropractic & Osteopathy 14(2), 4; Suehiro et al. (2015). Individuals with Chronic Low Back Pain Demonstrate Delayed Onset of the Back Muscle Activity during Prone Hip Extension. Journal of Electromyography and Kinesiology: Official Journal of the International Society of Electrophysiological Kinesiology 25(4), 675–80; Dwyer et al. (2013). Comparison of Gluteus Medius Muscle Activity during Functional Tasks in Individuals with and without Osteoarthritis of the Hip Joint. Clinical Biomechanics. 28(7), 757–61.

48. Yamato et al. (2015). Pilates for Low Back Pain. The Cochrane Database of Systematic Reviews, no. 7 (July), CD010265; Holtzman et al. (2013). Yoga for Chronic Low Back Pain: A Meta-Analysis of Randomized Controlled Trials. Pain Research & Management: The Journal of the Canadian Pain Society, 18(5), 267–72.

49. Petersen et al. (2014). Patellofemoral Pain Syndrome. Knee Surgery, Sports Traumatology, Arthroscopy. 22(10), 2264–74; Chester et al. (2008). The Relative Timing of VMO and VL in the Aetiology of Anterior Knee Pain: A Systematic Review and Meta-Analysis. BMC Musculoskeletal Disorders. 9(1), 64.

50. Lack et al. (2015). Proximal Muscle Rehabilitation Is Effective for Patellofemoral Pain: A Systematic Review with Meta-Analysis. British Journal of Sports Medicine 49(21), 1365-1376.

51. Willy et al. (2016). Current Concepts in Biomechanical Interventions for Patellofemoral Pain. International Journal of Sports Physical Therapy. 11(6), 877; Rabelo et al. (2018). Do Hip Muscle Weakness and Dynamic Knee Valgus Matter for The Clinical Evaluation and Decision-Making Process In Patients With Patellofemoral Pain? Brazilian Journal of Physical Therapy. 22(2), 105–109.

52. Willy (2016).

53. Willy (2016); Rabelo (2018).

54. Timmons et al. (2012). Scapular Kinematics and Subacromial-Impingement Syndrome: A Meta-Analysis. Journal of Sport Rehabilitation. 21(4), 354–70; Ratcliffe et al. (2014). Is There a Relationship between Sub- acromial Impingement Syndrome and Scapular Orientation? A Systematic Review. British Journal of Sports Medicine. 48(16), 1251–56. Struyf et al. (2013). Scapular-Focused Treatment in Patients with Shoulder Impingement Syndrome: A Randomized Clinical Trial. Clinical Rheumatology. 32(1), 73–85.

55. Struyf 2013; Camargo et al. (2015). Effects of Stretching and Strengthening Exercises, With and Without Manual Therapy, on Scapular Kinematics, Function, and Pain in Individuals with Shoulder Impingement: A Randomized Controlled Trial. The Journal of Orthopaedic and Sports Physical Therapy. 45(12), 984–97; McClure et al. (2004). Shoulder Function and 3-Dimensional Kinematics in People with Shoulder Impingement Syndrome before and after a 6-Week Exercise Program. Physical Therapy. 84(9), 832–48.

56. "A dynamic systems approach may provide a better framework for understanding." McQuade et al. (2016). Critical and Theoretical Perspective on Scapular Stabilization: What Does It Really Mean, and Are We on the Right Track? Physical Therapy. 96(8), 1162–69; Schellingerhout et al. (2008). Lack of Uniformity in Diagnostic Labeling Of Shoulder Pain: Time For A Different Approach. Manual Therapy. 13(6), 478-83.

57. Starrett (2014). Ready to Run: Unlocking Your Potential to Run Naturally, p. 60. Victory Belt Publishing.

58. Warr et al. (2014). Footstrike Patterns Do Not Influence Running Related Overuse Injuries in U.S. Army Soldiers. Medicine & Science in Sports & Exercise. 46, 812; Hamill et al. (2017). Is Changing Footstrike Pattern Beneficial To Runners? Journal of Sport and Health Science, 6(2), 146–153.

59. Gruber et al. (2013). Economy and Rate of Carbohydrate Oxidation During Running with Rearfoot And Forefoot Strike Patterns. Journal of Applied Physiology. 115(2), 194–201.

60. Hamill (2017); Hasegawa et al. (2007). Foot Strike Patterns of Runners at the 15-Km Point During an Elite-Level Half Marathon. Journal of Strength and Conditioning Research. 21(3), 888-893.

61. According to Hamill (2017): "changing to a mid or forefoot strike does not improve running economy, does not eliminate an impact at the foot-ground contact, and does not reduce the risk of running-related injuries."

62. Cavanagh et al. (1982). The Effect of Stride Length Variation on Oxygen Uptake During Distance Running. Medical Science and Sports Exercise. 14(1), 30-35; Hunter et al. (2017). Self-Optimization of Stride Length Among Experienced and Inexperienced Runners. International Journal of Exercise Science. 10(3), 446–53.

63. Dallam et al. (2005). Effect of a Global Alteration of Running Technique on Kinematics and Economy. Journal of Sports Sciences. 23(7), 757-64.

64. Schücker et al. (2018). Thinking About Your Running Movement Makes You Less Efficient: Attentional Focus Effects on Running Economy and Kinematics. Journal of Sports Sciences, 1–9.

65. Payne et al. (2016). Barefoot and Minimalist Running: The Current Understanding of the Evidence. Revista Española de Podología 27 (1). Consejo General de Colegios Oficiales de Podólogos: 1–3.

66. Neal et al. (2008). Foot Posture as a Risk Factor for Lower Limb Overuse Injury: A Systematic Review and Meta-Analysis. 85. Journal of Foot and Ankle Research. 7(1), 55; Nigg et al. (2015). Running Shoes and Running Injuries: Mythbusting and a Proposal for Two New Paradigms: 'Preferred Movement Path' and 'Comfort Filter.' British Journal of Sports Medicine. 49 (20), 1290–94.

67. Richter et al. (2011). Foot Orthoses in Lower Limb Overuse Conditions: A Systematic Review and Meta-Analysis—Critical Appraisal and Commentary. Journal of Athletic Training. 46(1), 103–6.

68. Baltich et al. (2015). Increased Vertical Impact Forces and Altered Running Mechanics with Softer Midsole Shoes. PLoS ONE 10(4), 1–11.

69. Nigg (2015).

70. Nigg et al. (2017). The Preferred Movement Path Paradigm: Influence of Running Shoes on Joint Movement. Medicine and Science in Sports and Exercise. 49(8), 1641-1648.

71. Mundermann et al. (2001). Relationship between Footwear Comfort of Shoe Inserts and Anthropometric and Sensory Factors. Medicine and Science in Sports and Exercise. 33(11), 1939–45.

72. Moran et al. (2017). Do Functional Movement Screen (FMS) Composite Scores Predict Subsequent Injury? A Systematic Review with Meta-Analysis. British Journal of Sports Medicine 51(23), 1661–69.

73. Lockie et al. (2015). Can Selected Functional Movement Screen Assessments Be Used to Identify Movement Deficiencies That Could Affect Multidirectional Speed And Jump Performance? The Journal of Strength & Conditioning Research. 29(1), 195-205; Okada et al. (2011). Relationship Between Core Stability, Functional Movement, And Performance. The Journal of Strength & Conditioning Research. 25(1), 252-261; Parchmann (2011). Relationship Between Functional Movement Screen and Athletic Performance. The Journal of Strength & Conditioning Research. 25(12), 3378-3384.

74. Frost et al. (2015). FMS Scores Change with Performers' Knowledge of the Grading Criteria-Are General Whole-Body Movement Screens Capturing 'Dysfunction'? Journal of Strength and Conditioning Research. 29 (11), 3037–44.

75. Tumminello et al. (2017). The Corrective Exercise Trap. Personal Training Quarterly, 4(1), 6–15.

CHAPTER ELEVEN: PAIN

1. Hoy et al. (2010). The Epidemiology of Low Back Pain. Best Practice & Research Clinical Rheumatology. 24(6), 769–781.

2. Chapman et al. (2008.) Pain and Stress in a Systems Perspective: Reciprocal Neural, Endocrine, and Immune Interactions. The Journal of Pain: Official Journal of the American Pain Society 9(2), 122–45; Abdallah et al. (2017). Chronic Pain and Chronic Stress: Two Sides of the Same Coin?" Chronic Stress (Thousand Oaks). 1, 10.1177/2470547017704763.

3. Melzack, Wall (1996). The Challenge of Pain, p.6. Penguin.

4. Recall the discussion in chapter four about how complex adaptive systems are often organized into different nested hierarchical levels. These relationships are similar to those seen in governments and businesses, where information and control can flow both "top-down" and "bottom-up."

5. Garland (2012). Pain Processing and the Human Nervous System: A Selective Review of Nociceptive and Biobehavioral Pathways. Primary Care - Clinics in Office Practice. 39(3), 561–71.

6. Reichling et al. (2009). Critical Role of Nociceptor Plasticity in Chronic Pain. Trends in Neurosciences. 32(12), 611–18; Price et al. (2015). Commonalities between Pain and Memory Mechanisms and Their Meaning for Understanding Chronic Pain. Progress in Molecular Biology and Translational Science. 131, 409–34.

7. Bove et al. (2003). Inflammation Induces Ectopic Mechanical Sensitivity In Axons Of Nociceptors Innervating Deep Tissues. Journal of Neurophysiology. 90(3), 1949–55.

8. This analogy has a view of sensory processing that is roughly similar to the theory of predictive coding. See, for example Clark (2013). Whatever Next? Predictive Brains, Situated Agents, and the Future of Cognitive Science. Behavioral and Brain Sciences. 36(3), 181–204.

9. Baliki et al. (2015). Nociception, Pain, Negative Moods and Behavior Selection. Neuron. 87(3), 474-91.

10. Woolf et al. (2011). Central Sensitization: Implications for the Diagnosis and Treatment of Pain." Pain. 152 (3 Supplemental), 1–31.

11. Woolf (2011).

12. Woolf (2011).

13. Price (2015).

14. It has been shown that if you expect a particular stimulus to be painful, this will increase the level of nociceptive firing in the spinal cord. Geuter et al. (2013). Facilitation of Pain in the Human Spinal Cord by Nocebo Treatment. Journal of Neuroscience. 33 (34), 13784–90.

15. Geva et al. (2017). Triathletes Lose Their Advantageous Pain Modulation under Acute Psychosocial Stress. Medicine and Science in Sports and Exercise. 49(2), 333–341.

16. Yarnitsky (2010). Conditioned Pain Modulation (The Diffuse Noxious Inhibitory Control-Like Effect): Its Relevance For Acute And Chronic Pain States. Current Opinion in Anaesthesiology. 23(5), 611–615; Fillingim et al. (2016). Assessment of Chronic Pain: Domains, Methods, and Mechanisms. Journal of Pain. 17(9), T10–T20. "Individuals with chronic pain often exhibit a pain modulatory imbalance, characterized by increased pain facilitation and diminished pain inhibition. This pattern has been observed for multiple pain conditions, including FM, temporo-mandibular disorders, irritable bowel syndrome, and osteoarthritis."

17. Melzack (2010). Pain and the Neuromatrix in the Brain. Journal of Dental Education. 65(12), 1378–1382.

18. This is called the "hard" problem of consciousness, a term coined by David Chalmers.

19. Moseley and Butler (2013). Explain Pain, 2nd Ed. NOI Group.

20. Fisher, et al. (1995) Minerva. BMJ 310, 70. https://doi.org/10.1136/bmj.310.6971.70

21. Moseley, et al. (2007). The Context of a Noxious Stimulus Affects The Pain It Evokes. Pain. 133(1-3), 64-71.

22. Höfle, et al. (2012). Viewing A Needle Pricking A Hand That You Perceive as Yours Enhances Unpleasantness Of Pain. Pain. 153(5).

23. Wand, et al. (2012). Seeing It Helps: Movement-Related Back Pain is Reduced by Visualization of the Back During Movement. Clinical Journal of Pain. 28(7), 602-8.

24. Stanton, et al. (2018). Illusory Resizing of the Painful Knee Is Analgesic in Symptomatic Knee Osteoarthritis. PeerJ. Jul 17, 6:e5206.

25. Ropero, et al. (2015). The Gate Theory of Pain Revisited: Modeling Different Pain Conditions with a Parsimonious Neurocomputational Model. Neural Plasticity. 4131395; Mendell (2013). Constructing and Deconstructing the Gate Theory of Pain. Pain. 155(2), 210-6.

26. Grahek, N. (2007). Feeling Pain and Being in Pain, 2nd edition. MIT Press.

27. Manchikanti et al. (2002). Understanding Psychological Aspects of Chronic Pain in Interventional Pain Management. Pain Physician. 5, 57–82; Leino et al. (1993). Depressive and Distress Symptoms as Predictors Of Low Back Pain, Neck-Shoulder Pain, And Other Musculoskeletal Morbidity: A 10-Year Follow-Up Of Metal Industry Employees. Pain. 53, 89–94.

28 Willoughby et al. (2002). The Effect of Laboratory-Induced Depressed Mood State on Responses to Pain. Behavioral Medicine. 28(1), 23–31; Tang et al. (2008). Effects of Mood on Pain Responses and Pain Tolerance: An Experimental Study in Chronic Back Pain Patients. Pain 138(2), 392–401.

29. Smith et al. (1998). The Meaning of Pain: Cancer Patients' Rating And Recall Of Pain Intensity And Affect. Pain. 78(2), 123–129.

30. Hechler et al. (2016). Why Harmless Sensations Might Hurt in Individuals with Chronic Pain: About Heightened Prediction and Perception of Pain in the Mind. Frontiers in Psychology. 7, 1638. For more on predictive pro-

cessing, see the book Surfing Uncertainty by Andy Clark, and this blog post I wrote on the subject: https://www.bettermovement.org/blog/2016/predictive-processing.

31. Benedetti, et al. (2011). How Placebos Change the Patient's Brain. Neuropsychopharmacology Reviews. 36, 339–354.

32. Marcuzzi, et al. (2018). From Acute to Persistent Low Back Pain: A Longitudinal Investigation Of Somatosensory Changes Using Quantitative Sensory Testing — An Exploratory Study. Pain Reports. 3(2), e641.

33. Marcuzzi (2018); Keedy et al. (2014). Health Locus of Control and Self-Efficacy Predict Back Pain Rehabilitation Outcomes. The Iowa Orthopaedic journal. 34, 158-65; Ahmed et al. (2019). The Effect Of Psychosocial Measures Of Resilience And Self-Efficacy In Patients With Neck And Lower Back Pain. Spine Journal. 19(2), 232-237.

34. Louw, et al. (2013). Neuroscience Education: Teaching Patients About Pain: A Guide for Clinicians. OPTP.

35. Patient education to improve self-efficacy is recommended for low back pain. Engers et al. (2008). Individual Patient Education for Low Back Pain. Cochrane Database Systematic Reviews. 2008; Louw et al. (2016). The Efficacy of Pain Neuroscience Education on Musculoskeletal Pain: A Systematic Review Of The Literature. Physiotherapy Theory and Practice. 32(5), 332-55. But note less hopeful findings in Traeger, et al. (2018). Effect of Intensive Patient Education vs Placebo Patient Education on Outcomes in Patients with Acute Low Back Pain. JAMA Neurology. 2018 Nov. 5.

36. De Heer, et al. (2014). The Association of Depression and Anxiety With Pain: A Study From NESDA. PLoS ONE. 9(10), 1–11.

37. Stubbs, et al. (2016). The Epidemiology of Back Pain and Its Relationship With Depression, Psychosis, Anxiety, Sleep Disturbances, And Stress Sensitivity: Data From 43 Low- And Middle-Income Countries. General Hospital Psychiatry. 43, 63–70.

38. Carnes (2007). Chronic Musculoskeletal Pain Rarely Presents in A Single Body Site: Results from A UK Population Study. May, 1168–1170; Tschudi-madsen, et al. (2011). A Strong Association Between Non- Musculoskeletal Symptoms and Musculoskeletal Pain Symptoms: Results from A Population Study. BMC Musculoskeletal Disorders. 18(12), 285.

39. Coggon et al. (2018). Drivers of International Variation In Prevalence Of Disabling Low Back Pain: Findings From The Cultural And Psychosocial Influences On Disability Study. European Journal of Pain. 23(1), 35-45.

40. Fibromyalagia is a controversial term. See, e.g. Yunus (2008). Central Sensitivity Syndromes: A New Paradigm and Group Nosology For Fibromyalgia And Overlapping Conditions, And The Related Issue Of Disease Versus Illness. Seminars in Arthritis and Rheumatism. 37(6), 339–352.

41. Clauw (2014). Fibromyalgia A Clinical Review. 311(15), 1547–1555.

42. Bradley (2009). Pathophysiology of Fibromyalgia. The American Journal of Medicine. 122(12 Suppl), S22-30; Chapman et al. (2010). Painful Multi-Symptom Disorders, a Systems Perspective. Chapter One of Translational Pain Research: From Mouse to Man. Kruger and Light, editors. Taylor and Francis.

43. Clauw (2014).

44. For a good summary of theories that view depression as a maladaptive and extreme form of psychological defense or "psychic pain" see the Wikipedia entry for "Evolutionary Approaches to Depression." https://en.wikipedia.org/wiki/Evolutionary_approaches_to_depression. For similar ideas about anxiety, see Bateson et al. (2011) Anxiety: An Evolutionary Approach. Canadian Journal of Psychiatry. 56(12), 707-15.

45. Blumenthal, et al. (2012). Opinion and Evidence: Is Exercise A Viable Treatment For Depression? ACSM's Health and Fitness Journal. 16(4), 14–21; Morres, et al. (2018) Aerobic Exercise For Adult Patients With Major Depressive Disorder In Mental Health Services: A Systematic Review And Meta-Analysis. Depression and Anxiety. 2018, 1–15.

46. Foster et al. (2018). Prevention and Treatment of Low Back Pain: Evidence, Challenges, And Promising Directions. The Lancet. 391(10137), 2368–2383.

47. Babatunde et al. (2017). Effective Treatment Options for Musculoskeletal Pain in Primary Care: A Systematic Overview Of Current Evidence. PLoS ONE. 12(6), 1–30.

48. The term "central" is a source of confusion because some use the term "central sensitization" to refer to a specific form of sensitivity at the dorsal horn, while others use it to describe a more generalized sensitivity to threat that

manifests in many different hierarchical levels of the nervous system, and other protective systems as well. I am using the word central in the latter sense.

49. Nijs et al. (2014). Applying Modern Pain Neuroscience in Clinical Practice: Criteria for the Classification of Central Sensitization Pain. Pain Physician. 17(5), 447-57.

50. Nijs (2014).

51. Nijs (2014).

52. There is a strong relationship between number of pain sites and overall health, sleep quality, and psychological health. Kamaleri et al. (2008). Number of Pain Sites Is Associated with Demographic, Lifestyle, And Health-Related Factors in The General Population. Europena Journal of Pain. 12(6), 742-8; Kamaleri et al. (2008). Localized or Widespread Musculoskeletal Pain: Does it Matter? Pain. 138(1), 41-6.

53. Phillips et al. (2011). Central Pain Mechanisms in Chronic Pain States--Maybe It Is All in Their Head. Clinical Rheumatology. 25(2), 141-54; Sarzi-puttini et al. (2011) Chronic Widespread Pain: From Peripheral to Central Evolution. Clinical Rheumatology. 25(2), 133–139.

54. Cook et al. (2016). Revisiting the Continuum Model of Tendon Pathology: What Is Its Merit In Clinical Practice And Research? British Journal of Sports Medicine. 50(19), 1187–1191.

55. Cook (2016); Rio et al. (2014). The Pain of Tendinopathy: Physiological or Pathophysiological? Sports Medicine. 44(1), 9–23; Rio et al. (2016). Tendon Neuroplastic Training: Changing the Way We Think About Tendon Rehabilitation: A Narrative Review. British Journal of Sports Medicine. 50(4), 209–215.

56. See chapter nine for various examples.

57. Consult the work of Jill Cook, Tom Goom, Peter Malliaris and Erik Meira for good practical information on finding the right level of intensity to load a tendon for rehab.

58. The least aggressive approach would be to try to move without provoking pain. This may not be possible, and research shows it may not be necessary. Exercise that creates some tolerable pain that doesn't get worse the next day is probably fine.

59. See Melzack et al. (2013). Pain. Wiley Interdisciplinary Reviews: Cognitive Science. 4(1), 1–15.

60. See, for example, the "protectometer" used by Butler and Moseley in *Explain Pain Protectometer*.

61. Flor (2002). Painful Memories. EMBO Reports. 3(4), 288–91.

62. Mansour et al. (2016). Chronic Pain: The Role of Learning and Brain Plasticity" Restorative Neurology and Neuroscience. 32(1), 129–139.

63. For examples, see the book *Pain Heroes* by Allison Sim. Also visit the blog of Joletta Belton at mycuppajo.com.

INDEX

A

adherence 27, 30, 104
affordance 106-109
agility 23, 177-179, 187
anxiety 38, 65, 80, 87, 202
attention 192
attractor 53-55, 173-175, 209-210
autoimmune disease 43, 80, 202

B

baby 4, 61, 156, 172
Bateson, Patrick 32
Bernstein, Nicolai 149, 161-171
biopsychosocial 10-11
Bosch, Frans 174
bottom-up 47, 56, 149, 163, 180
bracing the core 155
butterfly effect 50

C

catastrophizing 200
central sensitization 196
Chapman, Richard 201
chiropractor 128
climbing 38-39, 74-76, 106-7

complex adaptive systems 48-49
complicated (distinguished from complex) 58
coordination, defined 162
core strength 154-155
critical state 55, 210
Csikszentmihalyi M., 28, 33, 180

D

degrees of freedom 164-165
descending facilitation 197
descending inhibition 197
descending modulation 196
dexterity 162, 187
disc 120-121
dorsal horn 196
dynamic systems theory 161

E

ecological psychology 103
emergence 44-45, 61
endocrine system 30, 201-203
evolutionary mismatch 69
expectation 76, 200

F

fascia 127-128
feedback 50-54, 202
fibromyalgia 75, 202, 204
flow 28-29, 33, 180
fractal 43
Functional Movement Screen 186-187

G

Gibson, James 106
Goldilocks zone 72-73
Gretzky, Wayne 25

H

health, defined 10-11
HPA axis 68, 77, 202
hunter-gatherer 24, 39, 90, 93, 137, 151

I

illusions 199
immune system 46, 68-69, 75, 201
inflammation 51, 77-78, 195, 201, 209

J

just load it 184, 205

K

Kiely, John 77-78
kinesophobia 188

L

Lehman, Greg 184, 205
levels of motor control 166-170

M

McGill, Stu 114
Meadows, Donella 59
mechanoreception 199
Moseley, Lorimer 154, 196, 198
motivation, intrinsic 27
MRI 120-122
muscle knots 129

N

network 16-17, 47, 207
neuromatrix 198, 206-207
Newell, Karl 60
nocebo 188, 200
nociceptors 46, 195-196
non-linearity 49-50
nonlinear pedagogy 161
nutrition 5, 21, 86

O

obesity 68-69, 104
O'Sullivan, Peter 154-155

P

pain asymbolia 199
placebo 123, 200
Play
    and risk 34-38
    defined 27
    versus contest 31
Plsek, Paul 44, 58
PTSD 77, 202

R

reductionism 7, 42-43, 192
robust 38, 54, 56, 60, 119, 175
running 185-186

S

Sapolsky, Robert 69
self-efficacy 37, 105, 130, 200
self-organization 44, 55-56, 163, 167
Selye, Hans 70
sitting 23, 39, 94
sleep 75-76, 205-206
stretching 92, 138-139
subsystem 47
supersystem 47, 201
surgery 123-126

T

tendinopathy 204
Thelen, Esther 32, 116-117
top-down 47, 57, 60, 149, 157, 162, 180
trauma 46, 55, 76, 81, 195, 209-210

V

variability 44, 52-53, 96, 157, 163-164,
        174-175
vestibular 148

W

Watts, Alan 29
wicked problems 208
Wulf, Gabriel 179

Made in the USA
Monee, IL
07 October 2020

44243926R00142